"In a day when so much of the church exhibits a form of godliness but will not submit to His power, Ronnie Floyd, in *The Power of Prayer and Fasting: 10 Secrets of Spiritual Strength*, opens the door for many to experience afresh the supernatural power of an awesome God."

> H. B. London Jr., Vice President,
> Ministry Outreach/Pastoral Ministries,
> Focus on the Family

"Dr. Martyn Lloyd-Jones once asked, 'In these days of exceptional evil, are you doing something exceptional?' In this new book, Ronnie Floyd will challenge and equip you to do something exceptional for the kingdom of God. I encourage you to accept the challenge!"

> Dr. Steve Farrar, Men's Leadership Ministries

"Dr. Ronnie Floyd is a dynamic preacher, godly pastor, and an anointed leader. He practices what he preaches, and in this volume he is teaching what he has learned to practice. This book is not the theories of an armchair philosopher but the life and breath of a man on fire."

> Dr. Adrian Rogers, Pastor,
> Bellevue Baptist Church, Memphis, Tennessee

"One of the best books on prayer and fasting I've ever read. No matter who you are, your age, your profession or your spiritual goals, read, study, and take to heart Ronnie Floyd's 10 secrets to spiritual strength, and see your life changed forever."

> John C. Maxwell

"*The Power of Prayer and Fasting* reveals the true end of this neglected discipline: it is a gateway to intimacy with God; not an end in itself. It doesn't change circumstances or situations so much as it changes *us*. My dear friend Ronnie Floyd practices that which he preaches . . . and that makes this book worth reading, and reading again."

> Ed Young, Pastor
> Second Baptist Church of Houston

THE
POWER
OF
PRAYER
AND
FASTING

THE POWER OF PRAYER AND FASTING

10 SECRETS OF SPIRITUAL STRENGTH

RONNIE W. FLOYD

Foreword by Bill Bright

BROADMAN
&HOLMAN
PUBLISHERS

Nashville, Tennessee

A WORD OF CAUTION

Dr. Floyd is not a medical doctor. It is not the purpose of this book to advise you on the physical or medical aspects of fasting. *The Power of Prayer and Fasting* is written from a spiritual perspective and is based essentially on the author's personal experience. There are some individuals, because of medical conditions, for whom a fast would not be safe. Anyone considering a fast should assess his or her own physical condition and consult a physician familiar with fasting before beginning.

THE POWER OF PRAYER AND FASTING

Copyright © 1997 by Ronnie W. Floyd. All rights reserved. No portion of this book may be reproduced, stored in a retrieval system, or transmitted in any form or by any means—electronic, mechanical, photocopy, recording, or any other—except for brief quotations in printed reviews, without the prior permission of the publisher.

Published in association with Sealy M. Yates,
Literary Agent, Orange, California
Book Design by Kathryn Murray

Dewey Decimal Classification: 248.47
Subject Heading: Fasting \ Prayer
Library of Congress Card Catalog Number: 97-14644

Unless otherwise indicated, Scripture quotations used in this book are from the Holy Bible, New International Version (NIV). Copyright © 1973, 1978, 1984 International Bible Society. Used by permission of Zondervan Bible Publishers.

ISBN 1-56865-591-6

Printed in the United States of America

DEDICATION

I would like to dedicate this book to the ten thousand people of the First Baptist Church of Springdale, Arkansas. I dedicate it to each of you because you have prayed for me as God has developed His message in my life. Even though our relationship began a little over ten years ago, we both know that God has given you a new pastor over the last two years because of His work in my life through prayer and fasting.

I want to thank you, and tell you I love you very much because of your willingness to join God in what He is doing in my life and ministry. To God be the glory for the love relationship that He has given us as pastor and people. So with all my heart, I dedicate this book to you, my spiritual family called the First Baptist Church of Springdale, Arkansas.

CONTENTS

FOREWORD

THE BOOK IS A MAJOR MESSAGE of vast importance to God's people everywhere.

Dr. Ronnie Floyd combines his brilliant biblical insights and his profound experience with prayer and fasting to offer powerful, life-changing principles to every reader.

These principles can bring dynamic personal change, and they can bring national and world change, but these are not the most important potential effects. Far more importantly, these principles can help us to know our wonderful Lord better, more intimately, to draw nearer to Him, and to better experience His presence and power in our lives. And all these things, of course, help us to better glorify Him, to magnify Him with our lives, and to be more effective, fruitful vessels for Him to use.

During my fifty-three-year walk with our Lord, I had fasted many times—for one meal per day, one day per week, one week per month, and on one occasion for twenty-eight days. But it was not until 1994 that I experienced a forty-day fast. The blessings of the Lord exceeded my greatest expectations. Among other things, God used it to help bring more than six hundred Christian leaders together in Orlando, Florida in December of that year for three days of fasting and prayer, seeking the Lord, repenting and petitioning God for national and world revival and the fulfillment of the Great Commission. The very next month the media began reporting the breakout of revival fires on campuses and churches across the nation, and though there were other contributing factors, I strongly believe our fasting and prayer gathering made a very significant contribution to these revivals.

In 1995 I completed another forty-day fast, and the Lord brought 3,500 together in Los Angeles for Fasting & Prayer '95. The same thing happened in 1996, and approximately 4,000 gathered in St. Louis for Fasting & Prayer '96. As I write this foreward, I am beginning my fourth forty-day fast for revival for America, the world, and the fulfillment of the Great Commission. We anticipate hundreds of thousands possibly millions of God's people will participate live and via satellite across America from Dallas for Fasting & Prayer '97.

God seems to be building a powerful spiritual momentum for spiritual revival among His people. This wonderful book is part of that momentum.

Fasting with prayer is a spiritual atomic bomb in its potential power. Dr. Floyd shows you how to light the fuse. Prayerfully read, then prayerfully apply. You, and the world, will never be the same.

Dr. Bill Bright
Founder and President
Campus Crusade for Christ International

THE PREMISE AND THE PROMISE

A Preface

IMAGINE FOR A MOMENT that God might manifest His presence in your life in a powerful, unusual—even supernatural—way. Suppose He were to stand at your side, waiting to infuse your spirit with a fullness beyond your most cherished dreams or imagination. It would be a moment when God seems more real to you than at any time in your life. He would not be a God who cared one whit about *business as usual.* Instead, He would invite you to join Him in the most exciting, provocative, creative adventure of your life, promising you that He was ready, willing, and able to carry you into an experience so lofty, so eternally memorable, that you would never be the same.

Would you accept His generous offer? If so, you would discover that He suddenly would no longer be the former familiar *God in a box*—perhaps the God of your childhood on whom you called to scare away bogeymen, or to help find the penny you lost in the grass, or the Deity you prayed would prevent you from getting what may have been a well-deserved spanking. But now, in your adult imagination, He has become infinitely more than your childlike perceptions. Suddenly you sense He is watching you with His keen eyes, ready to engulf you with arms of love and His all-embracing heart . . . waiting, waiting. You sense He is almost pleading for you to enter His streams of blessing through a designated gateway that He has chosen for you. What should prevent you from entering that gateway? Asked more positively, what would be some of the reasons you would *choose* to enter that gateway?

In the midst of the mundane and mediocre, consider the excitement of being moved by God through being touched by something out of the ordinary. Imagine how shattered and dull the routine of an average day would be in the presence of your creative, loving heavenly Father—a God who chooses to take you by the hand and lift you higher than you've ever been lifted before. All with His generous promise that you would be energized by hope that your most desperate, fearful, confused moments would dissolve and dissipate in His presence.

The good news is that what I've just described is not a dream. This fresh experience with your heavenly Father can be yours. That's because God is still God. He is still on the throne. He hasn't changed, nor will He ever change. The God of the Bible is the same God who is waiting and willing to work in the lives of people like you and me today. The God of the universe who spoke worlds into existence, and who knows the number of grains of sand on every seashore, and who, if He chose to, could instantly calculate the number of hair follicles on our heads, wants to unleash His power on us.

REFRESHED BY THE FATHER

When this Lord of the universe comes to us, we can never be the same. He is not only the *waiting* Father but also our *approaching* Father. And as He comes toward us with His compelling vision for our better future, we find that circumstances, situations, things, and people begin to change. Mostly, *we* change. Yes, He's always been there, but now it all seems so different.

Strangely, when we are ready for His fresh, loving touch, God appears. He moves us off dead-center. Our small lives and shallow perspectives are challenged as we stand in awe of His holiness. The white heat of His holy presence penetrates our lives, and we are transformed. Once again, God works in ways that are out of the ordinary, defying natural explanation. His love is above and beyond anything we can think, imagine, or expect. His power is supernatural. It is beyond the natural, common, everyday experiences of our lives. The question is not, nor has it ever been, whether God is willing to move in the hearts of His people; the issue is whether we are willing to surrender in full obedience to Him so that we may begin to enjoy the enormous blessings He invites us to enjoy by living in His presence.

Times come when all Christians need fresh encounters with our loving God. Whether we become sidetracked by competing interests, or are overwhelmed by the struggles of life, we ultimately all drift from Him. That's why we need to reconnect with the Source of our being.

God is able and willing to bless His people in our day. He is waiting for individuals, churches, and nations to acknowledge their utter dependence on him and His grace. The bountiful spiritual blessings that He has promised will be showered on those who commit themselves to radical obedience and absolute trust.

While this book presents ten secrets that promise to lead to a deeper relationship with God, each is but one element in a singular, larger theme: *God's gateway to supernatural power can become ours when we come to our heavenly Father with contrite hearts and obedient spirits in fasting and prayer.*

ACKNOWLEDGMENTS

HOW CAN I SAY THANKS for all the things that God has done in my life through prayer and fasting? To God and God alone, I say, "Thank You for what You have done in my life through prayer and fasting. You have created the message in me for me to share in this book."

How can I say thanks to my research colleague, Robert C. Larson, who helped shape this material? He has been a friend, an encourager, and most of all a devoted brother in Christ. Thanks, Bob!

How can I say thanks to Broadman & Holman Publishers? During a seven-day fast in the fall of 1996, I asked God for a publisher who would not regard a book of this nature as just another book, but one who would have great conviction about its needed message to Christians in America and across the world. Broadman & Holman Publishers made a major commitment to this book. The people at Broadman & Holman believe with all their hearts that this message is needed across the world. Thank you to Ken Stephens and Bucky Rosenbaum for your strong support to this project.

How can I say thanks to my literary agents Sealy Yates and Tom Thompson? These men have placed each piece of the puzzle together. Thanks, Sealy and Tom.

How can I say thanks to Gayla Oldham, my excellent administrative assistant? She has felt the urgency for this book as much as I, and has made it high on her list of priorities. Thanks, Gayla!

How can I say thanks to my wife, Jeana, and my boys, Josh and Nick? During each extended fast, they made great sacrifices,

praying for me as God has developed His message in my life. They also sacrificed when countless hours were spent in writing a book. Thanks Jeana, Josh, and Nick!

How can I say thanks to the many people who have contributed to this book? Space will not permit me to give your names. Many of you were interviewed concerning the work of God in your own lives, in our church, and what you have sensed God has done in my life through fasting and prayer. You know who you are . . . thanks!

How can I say thanks to you who have decided to read this book? Enjoy the journey; thanks to all of you.

THE EXPECTATION AND THE EXPERIENCE

An Introduction

THE STORY YOU ARE ABOUT TO READ IS TRUE. The writer of the following letter is a Christian brother and friend. I am reproducing his letter early in this book because I want us to see what can happen when we are humbly obedient to God; when we choose to hear Him speak to us; when we determine to follow the path He sets for us. This brother's story will not be our story. We have our own lives to live, our own stories of joy and defeat to share, and our own daily, unique challenges to face. But this same God who continues to intervene in the life of the writer of this letter provides the same gateway to supernatural power to us. Please read his personal note to me, printed with his permission, in a spirit of worship and praise to a faithful, loving God.

Dear Pastor Floyd,

I want to take this opportunity to share what wonderful things God has been doing in my life and in the life of my family. I have felt led of God to tell you these things but am uncertain as to why. I trust that God knows, and that's good enough for me.

On Sunday, I completed my first extended fast. This was a totally new experience for me as I have never done anything remotely close to this in my lifetime. I would like to start by telling you how this all came about and then back up and give you a little history on myself.

About a year ago, I felt that God was asking me to move my family—my wife and two sons—to be part of your fellowship in Springdale, Arkansas. At that time it made absolutely no sense to do this because we were involved in our church and were very happy and comfortable there. At first, I discounted this feeling of "moving on" and went on with my life. However, the Lord kept bringing the issue to mind over and over again, and toward the summer, I found myself totally consumed with the idea of making the move. I finally gave in to God and visited your church on a Sunday evening (without my family). There was no more doubt. I knew that your fellowship was where my family and I needed to be. God did not reveal to me *why* we were to come, but He made it clear to me that we *must* come.

Breaking this news to my wife was like dropping a bomb on her. She resisted and fought me on this, and I began to wonder if our marriage was in trouble. I knew that I had heard a word from God but it seemed that my wife had lost all trust. She finally came, more out of compliance and to keep the family together than anything else. Once we started attending worship and Bible study, God demonstrated to us that we had made the right move.

Immediately, God started moving in me like nothing I've ever experienced in my life. I sensed He was calling me to fast. I resisted at first because fasting had always been a practice of legalism in my life in the past, and I didn't want even to consider fasting as a part of my spiritual life anymore. But God did not leave me alone on this issue either. It seemed like each day I was continually bombarded with the desire to fast.

I finally told God I would start fasting on January 1, and that I would fast for a short amount of time. This idea of a "short fast" lasted about two days. A fellow believer came and talked to a group of men I meet with regularly and discussed what God did for him when he fasted. I was deeply moved. He said he had lost a considerable amount of weight during this fast. I thought: *If I waited until New Year's Day to begin my fast, then people would just think I'd made another New Year's resolution to lose weight, and must really be doing a good job of it.* If this were to happen, all the attention would be on me and not on God! This is not what I wanted. I knew that fasting would have to be giving up physical food for a specific spiritual purpose. Somehow I found enough strength to commit to this fast. I must now give you a little history on myself.

This brother then begins to write about his formation, and how his life got started in the wrong direction—something he simply learned to endure.

When I was around nine years old, I was sexually abused by a boy in my neighborhood. This was just the beginning of years of abuse that followed. For some reason, I became involved with older athletic boys who provided physical protection for me at school in return for sexual favors. I didn't enjoy this at first, but eventually I learned to endure it. When I started growing and going through puberty, the abuse finally stopped. That's when I began to feel abandoned and unloved. I started masturbating on a daily basis, but this only brought me temporary comfort. I started looking at both heterosexual and homosexual pornography, and this provided only temporary satisfaction as well. A rumor got out at school that I was gay, and the majority of my guy friends left me. I realized I didn't fit in, and could hardly wait until the day I would move away to college.

My past came back to haunt me all the way through college—even into my married life. I actually started to believe that I was gay. So I thought, well if I were to get married, I couldn't possibly be gay. At first this idea worked. But after a couple of years of marriage, the desire to be with men started coming back. I knew then that I must be gay but would have to live a life of deceit to cover it up. I was in complete bondage to this and found myself falling back into old habits. I once again became involved with pornography. This time it was strictly homosexual in nature. I began to masturbate daily, and this kept me from wanting sexual relations with my wife. All of this was going on while I was involved in ministry. I couldn't believe that I could cover it all up so well.

Finally a close Christian brother noticed that something strange was going on. I confided in him that I was hooked on pornography, and I asked him to hold me accountable not to look at it again. I would have victory for a week and then fall again. I would always tell him that things were going great, knowing all the time this was simply another deception. I read many books about how to be set free, and even sought counseling, but nothing seemed to work. I was beginning to lose all hope. With that as background, and always so up front in my thinking, I began my fast.

One of the most important things to do prior to a fast is to ask God what He wants to accomplish during this intense time with him. That's why a prayer journal is so important. When you fast and pray, the prayers on your list *will be answered.* Brother "Z" made such a list.

I started listing several things that I wanted to ask God to work out in my life during this fast. Here is the list of my desires before God. I wanted:

- freedom from homosexual thoughts.
- freedom from pornography.
- to fall deeply in love with my wife again.
- to be a man of prayer.
- to be a humble person.
- freedom from gossip.
- financial freedom.
- to be able to know Christ in my life.

As I began to fast, I prayed that God would work a miracle in my life. I was amazed that, almost immediately, God delivered me from any desire to look at pornography or to masturbate. I knew that God would not be able to do anything in my life if these two things were present. Praise God, I experienced no withdrawals from these at all.

The next thing God starting working on was my pride and my very large ego. For a couple of weeks God showed me how there was too much of me in everything I did. I was always seeking the glory that belonged only to Him. I came to realize how I must have grieved the Holy Spirit so often. It was only when I repented of these sins that I sensed God was working mightily in me.

During my fast, I realized that God was also working in other areas of my life. He changed my heart to become a cheerful giver instead of a person who'd give out of obligation. I started noticing how my conversation was no longer filled with gossip. But the thing I started noticing most was how much I wanted to be with my wife, and how much I truly did love her. God was changing both of us, and the changes were allowing us to meet each other's needs. I find it hard to put these feelings into words, Pastor. I just know that my wife has captured my love, and I have captured hers.

Then, midway through the fast, once again I began having homosexual thoughts and dreams every day. I now honestly thought that there was no hope for my healing. I started getting very hungry about now and the thought of quitting the fast was ever-present. I spoke with my mother one evening and she encouraged me to quit, saying that God was probably finished showing me things. This didn't sit well with me, so I decided to pray for a renewed strength.

During this time of prayer is when the Holy Spirit started speaking to me. He revealed that the demonic oppression I was under would only stop through prayer and fasting. I had to complete the fast God called me to in order to be fully delivered from my affliction. That's when I realized my problem was with the demonic, and that the evil one wanted me to quit my fast. Satan was not about to relinquish any territory he had worked so hard to gain. Once I realized this, I was immediately filled with the presence of God and my strength was renewed.

I started noticing during the last week of the fast that my sinful, sordid dreams had stopped. Later I noticed that my thoughts were not slipping into anything homosexual in nature. It seemed as if I was experiencing God's victory hour by hour. On the last day of my fast, while writing in my journal, I realized that God really had set me free from the demonic stronghold of homosexuality! I was delivered! I was free! I was *clean!* From that moment on my life took on new meaning. I could think clearly, I could understand things that had baffled me before. The scales were removed from my eyes! *To God alone be the glory, great things He has done!*

Pastor, I share this with you because I know God wants me to. I give Him all glory and praise for what He has worked in me. I'm a new man today because of the healing power of God Almighty. I believe that prayer and fasting truly are the gateway to God's supernatural power.

Thank you for being obedient to God in sharing with us what our heavenly Father has instructed you to share. I pray that God will continue to sharpen me and lead me as I strive to serve Him with all I have.

With love and thanks to God,

"Z"

"Z" approached his time of fasting and prayer with the strong expectation that God would speak to him in ways he'd never been addressed before. His life was a complete mess: confused, misguided, and going nowhere. As you read in the letter, God did not leave him in his misery. He met "Z" at his greatest point of need, and this brother's life was transformed . . . and continues to be transformed today. One of my greatest joys in this book comes right now when I say that you, too, can enter that gateway to a supernatural experience with a living Savior—bringing your own needs, your own private concerns, and your own broken heart as you come into the holy presence of God.

O Lord, how many are my foes! How many rise up against me! Many are saying of me, "God will not deliver him."

PSALM 3:1–2

Your ways, O God, are holy. What god is so great as our God? You are the God who performs miracles; you display your power among the peoples.

PSALM 77:13–14

CHAPTER ONE
Knowing the Power of God

WE ENERGIZE OUR BODIES with power breakfasts and consummate important business deals over power lunches. We wear power ties of yellow and red, depending on our power taste. Our desktop computers are getting mini-er while providing us with more power than ever. The engines in our cars rev with more and more power. We read books that give us the 1, 2, 3s of achieving unlimited power. Self-help audio- and videotapes guarantee us all the power we'll ever need to be successful in business and in our personal lives. Power, power, power. But for all the promises made, and the vast number of good intentions laid out before us, someone invariably comes along and yanks on the plug, turns out our lights, and leaves us in darkness once again, forcing us to fend for ourselves as we go back to square one, defeated, out of gas, and powerless. Why do we do this to ourselves when the power of all power is only a prayer away?

Jesus proclaimed the power of His Father in some remarkable ways. One expression of His power was through *signs and wonders*. The laws of nature were temporarily put on hold as Jesus fed a mountainside of people with only five loaves of bread and two fish. A leper was made whole, to the surprise of everyone. Men of faith pulled away the tiles and lowered their disabled friend through a roof so Jesus could touch him and heal him. Lazarus was raised from the dead, an event to be followed later by the ultimate in death-defying feats—the resurrection of God's only Son. All of these were awesome and, you would think, convincing expressions of God's power.

In challenging the early church to embrace God's power, Paul often spoke about preaching that is effective not because of its human wisdom but because it is energized by the power of the Spirit of God. The core message of the New Testament is that the power of God changes lives, transforms points of view, and makes people new creatures. Power is a recurring theme throughout the Scriptures, but still, for many of us, we have only begun to understand the full ramifications of this power in our daily lives.

While we continue on our frantic search for the next promise of power, and yet one more *ultimate* in personal fulfillment, God stands at our side, patiently holding yet another connection that promises to link us with one of the greatest sources of power we will ever know. It's a source of power still underused, misunderstood, and even fear-evoking in the minds of some people. Purely and simply, it is the power of God that manifests itself through prayer and fasting.

MY JOURNEY

Although the discipline of prayer is frequently taught and practiced among Christians, the experience of knowing the power of God that comes through fasting, at least until recent days, seldom has been addressed in our generation. Even though fasting and prayer have been part of my life since my collegiate years, they have definitely taken on a new dimension in the past two years.

I have been active in the church most of my life, and have attended umpteen religious meetings and conferences over the years, but I cannot recall a single occasion when a call to fasting was given center stage. I don't remember ever receiving any instruction on fasting or what it could do for my spiritual walk. What little I did know, I picked up in my own study of God's Word. Early in my Christian experience, I made the decision to accept the Scriptures as the authoritative Word of God. As a result, what the Bible commands or teaches, I was determined to obey, even when I didn't understand its truth fully. It was through this commitment to biblical truth that I began to catch a tentative glimpse of the power of God that could and would become manifested in my life through fasting and prayer.

I have been active in the church most of my life, and have attended umpteen religious meetings and conferences over the years, but I cannot recall a single occasion when a call to fasting was given center stage.

I was a freshman in college when I first became fascinated with the many references to fasting in the Bible. I discovered that, by definition, fasting is *the abstinence from food with a spiritual goal in mind or for a spiritual purpose.* Well, if that's what God's Word said, I was prepared to believe it—and do it. Immediately, I made the commitment to one-, two-, and three-day fasts, all which became integral to my walk with God.

Fast-forward to Monday, January 15, 1990. My wife, Jeana, was diagnosed with cancer. I couldn't believe the news. My young, beautiful wife—with cancer? How could this be? I was desperate, and found myself truly powerless in dealing with the fear of not knowing what the future would hold. I knew I needed God's power at this difficult time in our family's life, and so I began fasting one day a week for forty weeks of the year. I'm not saying everyone should fast as I did, although I'm prepared to go on record as saying I know of nothing more powerful in my Christian experience. It has to be God's call, not ours. Fasting must be for a spiritual purpose, when we become so desperate for God that we have nowhere else to turn. And if God's command is to fast, then it's not an option.

At the end of that challenging, long period in our lives, God demonstrated His healing power, and today Jeana is free from that disease. That experience of God's power and presence was so authentic and life-changing for me that I continue to fast to this day. But God wasn't finished with me yet. Jeana's healing was as if I had only tasted of the Lord to see that He was good and faithful and trustworthy. There was much more to come.

In the spring of 1995, I felt God calling me to a fast of forty continuous days. On May 25, 1995, I concluded that fast. On May 9, 1996, I concluded my second fast of forty straight days. Only by God's grace, leadership, and power did I complete these days of fasting and praying—not for any glory to Ronnie Floyd, but as an act of worship to my all-powerful God who revealed His power to me again and again in ways I never thought possible.

Today, I write these words freely to demonstrate that my response comes from experience and deep personal conviction—my own personal pilgrimage—and is not motivated by a need to intellectualize the practice of fasting. Instead, as the sightless man whose only response to Jesus was, "Once I was blind, but now I see," so I, too, can say I have been changed inside and out. I am not the same man, the same preacher, the same husband, or the same father I once was. Fasting and prayer have been a gateway through which God has done supernatural things in my life, my family's life, and in my ministry. I have resolved that I will never face another major decision without first seeking the Lord's will and purpose through fasting and prayer. I am now also more convinced than ever that this miraculous gateway to God's supernatural intervention in the life of the believer is not exclusively reserved for a select few. It is the power of God available to everyone who trusts Jesus.

LOST IN THE WOODS

If your days are like mine, then we both know we all need frequent touches of God's presence and power. No Christian I know of is immune from this need for a renewed experience with our heavenly Father. We may not always be mindful of His presence as we become distracted by other interests. Too often we are so thrown by the struggles of our lives that we blunt our focus, turn to other *solutions*, and throw aside our compasses— our only hope for a way out. We're lost in the deep woods of despair, wondering if we'll ever find our way home. You've been there, and so have I. When we feel overpowered by our circumstances, intimidated by our challenges, and when we bleed over the pain of our wounds—an aching heart for relatives and friends who don't know Jesus, agony over illness that will not go away, palms wet with sweat as we worry about our economic future—our need for God becomes obvious. When we have exhausted our energy, watched our most carefully laid plans crumble around us, and have attempted every escape and remedy, the frailty of our fleshly existence meets us head-on. Whether it's an individual, a church, or a nation, we are nothing apart from our Creator and our created purpose. When the reality of who we are and who He is sets in, that's the time to give up, cry out in desperation, lift our hands, and place our hope in the only One who can save us. Without this reliance on God's power, we will be doomed to live half-lives, wallowing in mediocrity, never knowing the full joy of the Lord.

> ☀ When the reality of who we are and who He is sets in, that's the time to humble ourselves, cry out in desperation, lift our hands, and place our hope in the only One who can save us.

The good news is that God is able and willing to bless His people in our day with His unfailing supernatural power. He simply waits for individuals, churches, and nations to acknowledge their dependence on Him and His grace. Only then will the spiritual blessings He has promised be showered on those who commit themselves to radical obedience and absolute trust. But this won't come easily. There will be a price to pay.

REVIVAL WILL COME

This gateway to God's supernatural power is prayer and fasting. The Body of Christ must recognize these disciplines for what God has created them to be. Then I'm confident that a coast-to-coast, north-to-south spiritual revival will sweep across the United States and throughout the world when multitudes of Christians begin to engage in the spiritual disciplines of fasting and prayer. What is this revival? It is the manifested presence of God in our lives. It is when we allow our heavenly Father to be free to live in us, move us, and shape us into the image of His Son. In my first forty-day fast, the Lord confirmed in my heart that He was going to bring a mighty spiritual revival to America that promises to transcend all denominational, cultural, racial, and ethnic lines. Still, I realize that, for some, the word *revival* may have lost much of its coin because of overuse in religious circles. For many Christians, a *revival* has been reduced to an annual ritual or ecclesiastical event; a blip on a religious radar screen; an inconvenient interruption in an already over-scheduled week of lengthy, nightly meetings led by an out-of-town speaker on a local property owned by a zealous group of believers. That, for many, is revival.

This is not what I'm talking about in this chapter or in this book. True spiritual revival will transcend anything we have ever experienced. It will change the way we think about ourselves, our God, our present, and our future. It will alter the behavior of our neighbors and friends. True revival will come when God is taken seriously by those of us who call ourselves *followers of the Way*— who finally believe what we say we believe. True revival will be akin to spiritual seismic activity, shaking us to our core, allowing us to see the profound overtake the profane, with the promise that our lives will never be the same.

In his great novel, *Doctor Zhivago,* Boris Pasternak wrote two paragraphs that speak to what can happen to a culture when the Son of God manifests Himself in power and glory. This same God is still alive today, still standing at your side and mine, still ready and willing to open wide the gateway to the supernatural in the "new Rome" in which you and I live. The Russian author wrote:

> Rome was a flea market of borrowed gods and conquered peoples, a bargain basement on two floors, earth and heaven, a mass of filth convoluted in a triple knot as in an intestinal obstruction. Dacians, Herulians, Scythians, Sarmatians, Hyperboreans, heavy wheels without spokes, eyes sunk in fat, sodomy, double chins, illiterate emperors, fish fed on the flesh of learned slaves . . . all crammed into the passages of the Coliseum, and all wretched.
>
> And then, into this tasteless heap of gold and marble He came, light and clothed in an aura, emphatically human, deliberately provincial, Galilean, and at that moment gods

and nations ceased to be and man came into being—man the carpenter, man the plowman, man the shepherd with his flock of sheep at sunset, man who does not sound in the least proud, man thankfully celebrated in all the cradle songs of mothers and in all the picture galleries the world over.[1]

It happened before. It can—and will—happen again. This awakening will break the mold of all preconceived notions. It will rekindle the spirits and ignite the hearts of God's people. It will be exciting and dynamic. It will defy all human explanation. It will not be the exclusive product of any speaker or preacher, nor will be owned or controlled by any denomination, self-appointed group of believers, or spiritual clique. International borders will mean nothing. The coming revival will last longer than a week, will not be restricted to a tent with sawdust on the floor and hallelujahs echoing from the choir, and *for sure* it will interrupt much more than the evening's schedule of events. When it comes, we will know it, because it will be authentic and will spread like a raging fire in all directions. It could be as simple as a growing awareness of God's grace in our lives or as dramatic as a nation-wide—worldwide—awakening. This true revival will result in thousands, perhaps millions, of people saying yes to Jesus Christ. And it will bring the Body of Christ closer to fulfilling the Great Commission to go into all the nations and preach the gospel. If this is not the result of the awakening to come, then it will not be a revival at all.

The coming revival will last longer than a week, will not be restricted to a tent with sawdust on the floor and hallelujahs echoing from the choir, and *for sure* it will interrupt much more than the evening's schedule of events.

A WAKE-UP CALL FOR CHRISTIANS

The spiritual revival that God's people are now fasting and praying for will energize and motivate the entire Body of Christ. It will awaken America from its slumber. People from every walk of life, every culture, and every nation will come to know God's power. This true revival will shake our personal and corporate worlds. It will loosen the hinges of what we once thought was important. It will come to your life and mine when we quit *playing* church. It will come when we invite Jesus to be who He is and who He's always wanted to be in our lives.

How close are we to this occurrence? Closer than most of us realize, I feel. The power of God and the freshness of the Holy Spirit are everywhere. In some places it's only a spark. Elsewhere, it has already been fanned into a small flame. Through fasting and prayer this revival has already come to my life, and to the life of my congregation. Has this manifestation of God's power come to you? Are you going to sleep through the revival, or will you be a willing participant in the outpouring of God's power in the days to come?

ONE SPARK'S NOT ENOUGH

This true spiritual revival will sweep across the United States and the world when Christians begin to humble themselves and pray. Great numbers of believers throughout our land have already begun fasting and praying one, two, and three days at a time. Many have completed forty-day fasts. They are staff members in our churches, seniors, couples, single adults, college students, and even youngsters. All are coming to a new understanding of the power of God as they are called by God to fast and pray.

Years ago we sang a camp song with the words, *It only takes a spark to get a fire going.* I can tell you from personal experience that the spark of revival has now been ignited. But it's a big country and an even bigger world. One spark won't do it. This awakening will come only when the combined sparks of multitudes converge to create a conflagration of God's power.

Second Chronicles 7:14 says, "If my people, who are called by my name, will humble themselves and pray and seek my face and turn from their wicked ways, then will I hear from heaven and will forgive their sin and will heal their land." God wants to act on behalf of His people. But His actions are conditioned on the actions of His people. Humility in the presence of His power is what God demands of His children. Spiritual fasting is the *means*—the once-hidden, unexplored, misunderstood vehicle— by which we humble ourselves before God. If I knew of another way, I would preach it from morning to night. But I know of no other way to be humbled in His presence. Only when we come to our heavenly Father in His way and on His terms and respond according to His agenda will He unleash His bounty of blessing and pour out His reservoir of supernatural power on our lives.

HOW MUCH ARE YOUR SHOES PINCHING YOU?

Have you felt like quitting lately? Have you considered throwing in the towel and giving up, perhaps even on God, the church, and spiritual things? Have you even been so discouraged in your life you had to look up in order to see the bottom of your troubles? Have you ever felt things were so bad that it seemed as if God was shoving you up against the wall just to see what you were made of? Anyone who's honest would have to say "Yes, I've been there." But there's a much larger question that must be asked:

What do you *do* when you become desperate? Worry? Complain? Pray? Hope against hope that things will turn out right, that you'll get lucky, and that soon the dark clouds of despair will disappear from your seemingly doomed horizon? If, for some reason, you've not yet fallen into this pit of despondency, the less comforting news is that there *will* be times in your life when you will most definitely become desperate. But even this news is not all bad.

The word *desperation* implies that you will become frantic. You will feel rushed to make a decision—sometimes *any* decision. You will scurry about, looking for hope and searching for answers in the strangest places. You'll start asking God what in the world is going on. Your state of mind will affect every part of your being: spiritual, physical, social, and emotional. What do you do when you are desperate?

✳ Jehoshaphat knew that to fast before God was the best way to show his complete helplessness and humility before God. He learned something you and I must never forget: He renounced the natural to invoke the supernatural.

TAKING GOD SERIOUSLY

Second Chronicles 20:12 says, "O our God, will you not judge them? For we have no power to face this vast army that is attacking us. We do not know what to do, but our eyes are upon you." With enemy forces breathing down their necks, the people of Judah were in the thick of trouble. It looked as if it was going to be total devastation for God's anointed. Even Jehoshaphat, the warrior king, was afraid. He became so fearful that he turned all his attention toward seeking the Lord in his life as he began to pursue God more intently than he'd ever done before. In his terror at the prospect of massive defeat, the prophet proclaimed a fast throughout all of Judah. He asked the people to stop eating until God prevailed in their situation. He understood the spiritual practices of fasting and praying. Jehoshaphat knew that to fast before God was the best way to show his complete helplessness and humility before God. He learned something you and I must never forget: He renounced the natural to invoke the supernatural.

He declared, "God, I don't want food, I want You. You are more important than food." This was not a popular theme then any more than it is a driving principle in the hearts of large numbers of believers today. But it *is* a principle. It's a *revival* principle—a *resurrection* principle, and a resurrection always is most credible in a graveyard—an apt word for much of what we see in today's world. The secular humanism and worldliness that is infiltrating the church and encroaching on our lives doesn't ask us to call on God for His strength and power. Not by a long shot.

The world keeps on telling us to be more positive about who we are: "Live up to your potential. You can do it! See the glass as half-full, not half-empty. If it is to be, it's up to me! Every day and in every way things are getting better and better." Really? I hadn't noticed. This kind of thinking can derail us when we allow the spirit of Madison Avenue and the misguided counsel of most of the self-help gurus of the motivational circuit to subvert the Spirit of the living God. We really *do* believe that whoever ends up with the most toys wins. We want our cake, our pie, our cars, our bank accounts, our stocks and bonds, our steak, and our mashed potatoes with gobs of gravy more than we are willing to feast on the bountiful riches of our heavenly Father. But when we're desperate, *we cannot have it both ways.* The toys have to go, along with anything else that puts a barrier between us and God. The truth is this: We are powerless in and of ourselves. And because physical food is not our ultimate source of nourishment, then physical food must be seen in its physical perspective: We, like the prophet, must be willing to renounce the natural to invoke the supernatural.

FREEDOM AT LAST

Jehoshaphat proclaimed a fast for his people *so they could once again see the face of God.* He said that they sought Him and kept their eyes on Him. When they became desperate, they shifted their focus to God and away from their hopeless, degenerate, discouraging, depraved situation. It was their choice, and it's also ours. When we become desperate enough, we, too, will drop to our knees, seek the Father, and keep our eyes fixed on Him, with the knowledge that one of the gateways to His supernatural intervention in our lives is through fasting and prayer.

When we are delivered from our despair by removing our focus from food to spending time with God, something takes place in our hearts that we can't control. Our spirits bear witness with the Spirit of God. Suddenly we say, "It's happened. God has finally stepped into my life. I've been delivered. I'm free. I've tapped into God's power in a supernatural way." Then something else amazing happens. Rather than getting on the phone to talk about the ball game or the latest rise or fall in stocks, we find ourselves saying, "Mary . . . Joe, I can't believe what God is doing in my life, and I just had to tell somebody." That's what it means to worship and praise our living God.

God wants us to be conscious of His presence. He wants to give us hope for the present and confidence in our future. He wants to give us an attitude of thanks that we've never had before. He wants to do something mighty in our lives, and that's why He provides us with moments of desperation—to push us toward Him. Who is in charge of our desperate moments? God. Nothing happens to us that does not come first through His strong yet gentle hand. God is eternally up to something, and we can count on it. When we become desperate, it will always be for a reason. It means God is speaking to us. He wants our undivided attention. He's demanding our uncomplicated allegiance. To have His way with His *always-hungry* followers, He reminds us to pause often in His presence, remove the physical food from our table, and replace it with the bread that satisfies eternally, along with the nurturing water of the Spirit that promises us we will never thirst again.

OUR STRENGTH—A MIRAGE IN THE DESERT

Even a limited understanding of our human condition should persuade us that to be wise is to reject the utter arrogance of personal sufficiency. We don't have what it takes to *go it alone*. Our strength is a mirage that makes a mockery of our intentions, even as the water hole that doesn't exist creates delirium in the mind of a deluded desert traveler. We don't need God's supernatural power as an add-on to our own. That's the spiritual equivalent of mixing oil and water. We need His power and strength because we are so infinitely sinful and weak. Still, with our mixed bag of misguided motives and frailties, the church of Jesus Christ is a sleeping giant, its unrealized capacity to be God's vehicle for true revival almost too staggering to imagine. What remains is a need for that incendiary fellowship of dedicated, committed men, women, and children who will trust God to be God, who will not settle for ho-hum religion, and who will enter with joy the gateway to His supernatural power through the God-ordained vehicles of fasting and prayer.

And so we travel on, called to be enlisted in a growing army of believers who serve the King of Kings. We've been granted the eternal promise that when we wait on the Lord our strength will be renewed, we'll run and never feel tired, walk and not faint. Our renewal is in Him, and for this reason we can be assured that a spiritual awakening is at hand—revival that starts in your heart and mine. The truth is this: Life is not about food on the table. It *is* about eating the Bread of Life that promises eternal satisfaction— and eating it *humbly in the presence of our heavenly Father*—the second secret in our discovery of God's gateway to supernatural power.

Some became fools through their rebellious ways and suffered affliction because of their iniquities.

PSALM 107:17

He guides the humble in what is right and teaches them his way. All the ways of the LORD *are loving and faithful for those who keep the demands of his covenant.*

PSALM 25:9–10

CHAPTER TWO
Coming Humbly Before God

HUMILITY! We've all heard the story of the person who allegedly wrote the book *Humility and How I Attained It* (now available in five volumes)! We laugh at this apocryphal volume for good reason: Humility is tough. Unnatural. It goes against an insidious self-worship that's integral to our lives. We take pride in our looks, our accomplishments, the cars we drive, the money we make, and the houses we live in.

Unfortunately, our lack of humility doesn't stop there. We're often even prouder of how we live our Christian walks thinking, "No one reads the Bible as much as I do. No one is as active in church as I am. I'm a pillar of our congregation, and they'd know it in a heartbeat if I weren't Johnny on the spot." Hardly the thoughts of humility. It reminds me of the English vicar who had six of his academic degrees painted on the glass door that led to his study. Underneath these symbols of decades of scholastic achievement were the words, "Your humble servant. Please make an appointment with my secretary."

While the Scriptures urge us on to perfection, they give us no encouragement to suppose that perfection will ever be achieved as long as we occupy this mortal flesh. Those of us who think for even a moment that we are righteous are not righteous at all. For this reason, we are afflicted with a terminal disease called spiritual pride, the most deadly manifestation of our sinful nature.

But what does it mean to be humble before God? Why is it important that we lower our estimate of ourselves in prayer and fasting before our relationships with God can move to a new level?

GOD'S WORD ON THE SUBJECT

Sometimes we may be reading the Bible too selectively, and in the process forget what God's Word has to say to us on the subject of being humble before Him. But when we take the time to search for God's truth in this matter, we read:

- But Gideon told them, "I will not rule over you, nor will my son rule over you. The LORD will rule over you." (Judges 8:23)

- This is what the LORD says: "Let not the wise man boast of his wisdom or the strong man boast of his strength or the rich man boast of his riches." (Jeremiah 9:23)

- Then King David went in and sat before the LORD, and he said: "Who am I, O Sovereign LORD, and what is my family, that you have brought me this far?" (2 Samuel 7:18)

- Now, O LORD my God, you have made your servant king in place of my father David. But I am only a little child and do not know how to carry out my duties. (1 Kings 3:7)

- The LORD is close to the brokenhearted and saves those who are crushed in spirit. (Psalm 34:18)

- Better is one day in your courts than a thousand elsewhere; I would rather be a doorkeeper in the house of my God than dwell in the tents of the wicked. (Psalm 84:10)

- I baptize you with water for repentance. But after me will come one who is more powerful than I, whose sandals I am not fit to carry. He will baptize you with the Holy Spirit and with fire. (Matthew 3:11)

- For whoever exalts himself will be humbled, and whoever humbles himself will be exalted. (Matthew 23:12)

- Humble yourselves before the Lord, and He will lift you up. (James 4:10)

- If my people, who are called by my name, will humble themselves and pray and seek my face and turn from their wicked ways, then will I hear from heaven and will forgive their sin and will heal their land. (2 Chronicles 7:14)

OUR MIDNIGHT CRISIS

Saint Augustine wrote, "Do you wish to be great? Then begin by being. Do you desire to construct a vast and lofty fabric? Think first about the foundations of humility. The higher your structure is to be, the deeper must be the foundation." It is no great accomplishment to be humble when the circumstances of life bring us to our knees. But to choose a humble spirit when we are praised is a rare occurrence—and impossible in our own strength. This is why we have no alternative but to walk through the gateway to supernatural power with heads bowed low in humility before our Creator God—*the gateway of fasting and prayer.*

Because of the surrounding cacophony that screams, demands, and cajoles us to do our own thing, we need a clear, uninterrupted message from God to stay on course. The spiritual vital signs in this nation, in our churches, and in our individual lives display our desperate need for a word from God that hits us between the eyes, takes the wind out of our self-importance, reminds us that we are *not* God, and brings us to our knees. Why? Because we are living in a midnight crisis, and unless we humble ourselves with fasting and prayer, we will not know real joy, we will not know God's best for our lives, and we will never experience personal or national revival.

※ **The answer to our spiritual crisis will not be found in the ballot box but in the prayer closet. The answer to our personal and corporate dilemma will not come through high-tech, hyperbole, and hype.**

As we race toward the coming millennium, we need to stop long enough to evaluate where our country is, where our churches are, and where *we* are. Would anyone question that we live under ominous clouds of spiritual darkness? Unless we bow humbly before our God, that cloud will become even thicker, and the Body of Christ will find itself increasingly immobilized, unable to support itself because of its own dead weight.

The answer to our spiritual crisis will not be found in the ballot box but in the prayer closet. The answer to our personal and corporate dilemma will not come through high-tech, hyperbole, and hype. It *will* come through a fresh touch from our heavenly Father who wants to speak to us, move us, and shower us with His mighty presence. The answer to our spiritual malaise will not come through the restructuring of our denominations, appointing more standing committees, and having more conventions, although these have their place. The answer to our spiritual crisis will come when we put off our mind-sets of self-worship, territorialism, and the spirit of arrogance and pride, and put on the sackcloth of prayer and fasting and humiliation and repentance before God.

AMERICA'S SPIRITUAL CRISIS

Today, three out of four Americans don't believe in absolute truth. This simply means that most don't believe that any one thing is either right or wrong, but that truth lies hidden somewhere in a distant fog, unexplainable and unimportant. For these individuals, there is no such horrific thing as sin, nothing that comes close to judgment, and therefore, obviously, what a silly idea it is that we should ever need a Savior. He would be a contradiction in terms.

Because we have veered so far off course, it should not seem surprising that we are seeing an escalation of teen pregnancy and a dramatic increase in abuse perpetrated on the innocent by people from all walks of life. More than 3 million children are abused each year, 1.3 million sexually. Integrity is quickly becoming an unknown word. Approximately $6 billion each year is thrown away on state-approved and illegal betting. We spend $10 billion each year polluting our bodies with tobacco products. Some 10 million drink themselves into oblivion every day in this nation. Cybersex on the Internet is now entering our homes at an alarming rate, appealing to the prurient interest of those with computers, with our children logging on in increasing numbers. At the same time, we are watching the homosexuality movement continue to infiltrate our lives and even determine much of our country's future agenda. As we see the rate of abortion—and now the *ending of life* by someone referred to as "Dr. Death"—it's all the more important that we understand that we are stuck in a major spiritual crisis.

CRISIS IN OUR CHURCHES

But there's another issue that doesn't make it into the headlines. It's the spiritual crisis in our churches. Most of our mainline churches have either plateaued or are declining. What is the problem? For one thing, we're turning minor concerns into major issues. We are not spending our time talking about justice, mercy, humility before God, and becoming His faithful servants. Instead, the typical major issues in our churches today are, "Should we clap in church?" "Should we sing choruses or hymns?" "Do we project the words of our songs onto large video screens, or do we use hymnbooks?" "Do we have a praise band or a choir? And, oh, do they wear robes or regular clothes?" It makes me think of what Jesus said to the overly righteous, out-of-touch, stuck-in-tradition Pharisees. He pulled no punches as He spoke in some of the strongest language He ever used:

> Woe to you, teachers of the law and Pharisees, you hypocrites! You give a tenth of your spices—mint, dill and cummin. But you have neglected the more important matters of the law—justice, mercy and faithfulness. You should have practiced the latter, without neglecting the former.
>
> You blind guides! You strain out a gnat but swallow a camel.
>
> Woe to you, teachers of the law and Pharisees, you hypocrites! You clean the outside of the cup and dish, but inside they are full of greed and self-indulgence. Blind Pharisee! First clean the inside of the cup and dish, and then the outside also will be clean.
>
> Woe to you, teachers of the law and Pharisees, you hypocrites! You are like whitewashed tombs, which look beautiful

on the outside but on the inside are full of dead men's bones and everything unclean. In the same way, on the outside you appear to people as righteous but on the inside you are full of hypocrisy and wickedness.

Woe to you, teachers of the law and Pharisees, you hypocrites! You build tombs for the prophets and decorate the graves of the righteous. And you say, "If we had lived in the days of our forefathers, we would not have taken part with them in shedding the blood of the prophets." So you testify against yourselves that you are the descendants of those who murdered the prophets. Fill up, then, the measure of the sin of your forefathers!

You snakes! You brood of vipers! How will you escape being condemned to hell? Therefore I am sending you prophets and wise men and teachers. Some of them you will kill and crucify; others you will flog in your synagogues and pursue from town to town . . . I tell you the truth, all this will come upon this generation.

O Jerusalem, Jerusalem, you who kill the prophets and stone those sent to you, how often I have longed to gather your children together, as a hen gathers her chicks under her wings, but you were not willing. Look, your house is left to you desolate. For I tell you, you will not see me again until you say, "Blessed is He who comes in the name of the Lord." (Matthew 23:23–39)

Can you relate to these hard words of Jesus? If you're like me, you can actually feel your flesh crawl when reading: "You are like whitewashed tombs, which look beautiful on the outside but on the inside are full of dead men's bones and everything unclean. In the same way, on the outside you appear to people as righteous but on the inside you are full of hypocrisy and wickedness." I read this with a broken heart and I say, "Ronnie Floyd, that's you. You've been so proud, so self-centered, parading your gifts so all could see them, so eager to make a name for yourself. You are really nothing but a stinking, rotten tomb, full of dead bones, hypocrisy, and wickedness."

But that's not the kind of man, pastor, father, and husband I *want* to be. I want God's best. I want to fight the right battles on the right battlefront with the right weapons. I want to know what price God wants me to pay for a life of holiness, and I am prepared to pay that price. It took me a long time to understand this, but I now have gotten a glimpse of the eye of the Father, and He has ushered me through His gateway to supernatural power.

WHERE HAS ALL THE LEADERSHIP GONE?

What has happened to the real issues in our churches—issues such as personal growth in Christ, community witnessing, and world evangelization? What has happened to issues such as reconciliation and repentance? What has happened to our preaching on prayer and fasting and personal awakening to God's best? Why are we not reaching our young people in more effective ways? Without these issues being center stage, how can there ever be revival in our hearts and in our land?

While 70 percent of the advertising budgets of many secular companies targets teenagers, selling them everything from makeup to porn, the average church in this country allocates less than 2 percent of its budget to reach the next generation for Jesus Christ. If this doesn't change, we are going to wake up one day and discover we're preaching to those who have only gray hair or no hair.

We may have people who wear the label of inerrancy on their shirt pocket rather than the label of moderate, but if this is our only focus, we will soon become a nation of churches filled with old wineskins—brittle, inflexible, without life, and useless. As we see the dawning of a new millennium, there is no question that we are in a major midnight spiritual crisis.

While 70 percent of the advertising budget of many secular companies targets teenagers, selling them anything from makeup to porn, the average church allocates less than 2 percent of its budget to reach the next generation for Jesus Christ.

OUR CRISIS—A RERUN OF HISTORY?

But what does the Bible say about this crisis? Has humanity ever been here before? Of course it has. It's what the prophets themselves were most concerned about. It's the nature of our human condition when we go our own way, make our own rules, and put God on a shelf for a day *when we might need him.* God's people in Judah were in a spiritual crisis continually. On one occasion, drought and locusts served as God's judgment on their sin. The devastation was so great in the land that the people could not even offer grain offerings to the Lord. Their only hope was repentance. Enter the prophet Joel who called the people of God to repent of their sin. That call is for you and me to humble ourselves, pray, fast, and repent during this midnight hour. Why? So, as we stand on the threshold of a new millennium, we might experience a deep, life-changing moving of the Spirit of the living God in our lives.

Key spiritual principles in the Book of Joel are apropos to our self-centered lives today. As our spiritual lives go, so go the spiritual lives of the leaders in our families, our churches, and in our nation. Every one of us is a leader because we have influence over *someone*. We are either fathers, mothers, pastors, teachers, uncles, aunts, brothers, or sisters. In some area of your life *you are a role model—a person of influence*. The question is: How well are you doing in your role? How is your influence being felt? Is it for good or for ill?

MODELING BROKENNESS

To enter God's gateway to supernatural power, you and I must model spiritual brokenness, humility, and repentance before the people of God and the world in which we live. Some things may be the worse for breaking, but a heart is never at its best until it is broken by the things that break the heart of God. Are we modeling this brokenness and repentance? Our answers will indicate the power of our spiritual lives. Hear the word of the Lord from Joel 1:9–20—a passage that speaks as confidently today as it did when God spoke it with power through His servant.

> Grain offerings and drink offerings are cut off from the house of the LORD. The priests are in mourning, those who minister before the LORD.
>
> The fields are ruined, the ground is dried up; the grain is destroyed, the new wine is dried up, the oil fails.
>
> Despair, you farmers, wail, you vine growers; grieve for the wheat and the barley, because the harvest of the field is destroyed. The vine is dried up and the fig tree is withered; the pomegranate, the palm and the apple tree—all the trees

of the field—are dried up. Surely the joy of mankind is withered away.

Put on sackcloth, O priests, and mourn; wail, you who minister before the altar. Come, spend the night in sackcloth, you who minister before my God; for the grain offerings and drink offerings are withheld from the house of your God.

Declare a holy fast; call a sacred assembly. Summon the elders and all who live in the land to the house of the LORD your God, and cry out to the LORD.

Alas for that day! For the day of the LORD is near; it will come like destruction from the Almighty. Has not the food been cut off before our very eyes—joy and gladness from the house of our God?

The seeds are shriveled beneath the clods. The storehouses are in ruins, the granaries have been broken down, for the grain has dried up. How the cattle moan! The herds mill about because they have no pasture; even the flocks of sheep are suffering.

To you, O LORD, I call, for fire has devoured the open pastures and flames have burned up all the trees of the field. Even the wild animals pant for you; the streams of water have dried up and fire has devoured the open pastures.

WAKE UP, AMERICA!

We are in the same condition as God's people during the time of the prophet Joel. The time has come to respond to the alarm. It's time for America to wake up, just as the priests and the ministers of the Lord in Joel's day were shaken out of their sleep over the sinfulness of Judah. If we are to know God's supernatural power, we, too, must have spirits that are contrite and broken. It broke the priests' hearts that they could not make any offering at all to God. God's judgment had been so mighty *that there was nothing left to offer.* They wept and wailed before the God of heaven. They humbled themselves through fasting. They demanded national repentance by calling for a solemn assembly to cry out to the Lord. Their tears were expressions of honest grief, and in their pain they interceded for the people of God. How broken are we today? In Jesus, *we* fulfill the role as a kingdom of priests.

※ **It broke the priests' hearts that they could not make any offering at all to God. God's judgment had been so mighty *that there was nothing left to offer.***

How do you read this passage from Joel? Do you see it as another fascinating, but perhaps ho-hum, history of an ancient people who never seemed to be able to get it together spiritually? Or do you read these verses as a prophetic rendering of where you live today? If we take God's Word at face value, then these words from Joel *will* do something to challenge our hearts to take action.

They must touch us, break us, and drive us to a new desire to know God. When was the last time we were broken with grief over our own sins and alienation from our heavenly Father? When was the last time we confessed with tears that we were playing church games—just showing up so we could show off, while we knew we were little more than a sordid display of dead men's bones? When did we last intercede on behalf of our bosses, our colleagues at work, or the members of our own families with sorrowful hearts? When was the last time we fasted and prayed over our own spiritual plights, the spiritual conditions of our churches, and the spiritual health of our country? When was the last time we sensed God's calling us to repent of *anything*, especially our separation from the God who made us, loves us, and gave His Son for our eternal souls? When was the last time we were consciously willing to submit to His leadership, and willfully turn from sin when He called us to repent? When was the last time we called for a solemn assembly to cry out for God to forgive us and our brothers and sisters from our sins of racial prejudice, greed, lust, love of material things, and anything else that stands between us and God?

YOU ARE A LEADER

Have we ever been so humbled that we could hardly absorb the presence of God because we knew we were standing on holy ground? In our roles as leaders—and please remember, *we are all leaders*—have we ever been bold enough, tenacious enough, and spiritually concerned enough, to weep at the altar, asking God to bring a mighty spiritual awakening to our lives, and to the lives of those around us? If we don't model spiritual humility born from our own deep experiences with God, if we don't model spiritual brokenness, and if we don't model repentance from our self-centeredness and demand for control, we will never see a spiritual awakening in our own lives or in the life of our nation.

As we exercise our spiritual gifts, and direct others to this gateway to supernatural power, we will be on our way to personal and national revival. God's people are the keys to this awakening in our time. It doesn't matter what the left-wing liberal does, and it doesn't matter what the right-wing says. Denominations may have things to contribute—they'll always have things to contribute—but their discourses ultimately won't be all that important. All that matters is what we, the people of God, do about our own spiritual conditions.

Joel 2:12–13 says, "'Even now,' declares the LORD, 'return to me with all your heart, with fasting and weeping and mourning. Rend your heart and not your garments. Return to the LORD your God, for he is gracious and compassionate, slow to anger and abounding in love, and he relents from sending calamity.'"

FASTING AND PRAYER ARE NOT OPTIONAL

The command of God is laser clear: The people of God are to return to him humbly, with their whole hearts—with fasting, weeping, and mourning. We may not like to hear those hard words of God. Perhaps we'd like to come back to God on other terms, when it's a more convenient time, when the price is not quite so high, when God changes His mind, when we can continue with a spirit of business as usual, and when we won't have to change our present thinking about God or His kingdom. I'm afraid none of those is even a remote option. What God demands of us is not up for debate. We must enter the Father's presence one way only—humbly, with our whole hearts, grieving for our sins, and with prayer and fasting. It is neither a prerogative nor luxury to suggest compromises when God has told us what is necessary for us to return to Him.

This is God's gateway to supernatural power—a power we will ultimately employ if we are to survive our spiritual dilemma.

But more than survival, this power will manifest itself with a mighty, refreshing, heart-changing revival of the Holy Spirit upon individuals and the church in the midst of our midnight crisis.

※ We must come to our heavenly Father only one way—humbly with our whole hearts, grieving for our sins, and with prayer and fasting. It is neither our prerogative nor luxury to demand compromises when God has told us what is necessary for us to return to Him.

Q: *What will happen when we allow almighty God to be ruler of our lives?*

A: "Then, the LORD will be jealous for his land and take pity on his people" (Joel 2:18).

Q: *What will God do on our behalf?*

A: "The LORD will reply to them: 'I am sending you grain, new wine and oil, enough to satisfy you fully; never again will I make you an object of scorn to the nations" (Joel 2:19).

Q: *What will be the tangible results in the lives of those who trust and fear God?*

A. Joel 2:28–32 says, "And afterward, I will pour out my Spirit on all people. Your sons and daughters will prophesy, your old men will dream dreams, your young men will see visions. Even on my servants, both men and women, I will pour out my Spirit in those days. I will show wonders in the heavens and on the earth, blood and fire and billows of smoke. The sun will be turned to darkness and the moon to blood before the coming of the great and dreadful day of the LORD. And everyone who calls on the name of the LORD will be saved; for on Mount Zion and in Jerusalem there will be deliverance, as the LORD has said, among the survivors whom the LORD calls."

THE NEXT GREAT MOVE OF GOD

When God's people repent in humility and desperation, and when we return to Him with our whole hearts, God will bring a true awakening just prior to the second coming of our Lord. God says He will do mighty, miraculous works. He will demonstrate His power with supernatural things in our midst, but only if we return to him with our whole hearts. There is no other way. The exam is not multiple choice. And the fulfillment of this passage from Joel will not occur until moments before the return of Jesus Christ. How close is this day?

A large part of the answer lies in our own hearts and minds: How serious are we about returning to God with our whole hearts, humbly asking His will for our lives? When the awakening does come, we will see God do things we have never observed before. He will unleash a power unknown to us or anyone who came before us in human history. We will experience a touch from God that will shake us individually, shake this country, and shake this world. It will move the gospel of Christ across the globe faster than a signal from CNN and at greater speeds than the latest NASA rocketry. It's past time to strip off the garment of the skeptic. It's time to remove the mentality of the critic. It's time to eliminate the perverse thinking of the jealous. It's time to shed the skins of the proud and the arrogant.

If we are going to come to *Him*, we must get on *His* ground, operate on *His* terms, and let God do what God wants to do.

God is moving in a great way, and it's important that we realize He will move with or without us. But because He is our loving

Father, He wants us to make the right choice—to go His way, to do His bidding, to be His children. Our God does not need us; we need Him. So it follows that if we are going to come to *Him*, we must get on *His* ground, operate on *His* terms, and let God do what God wants to do.

THE STAGE IS BEING SET

If God does not step into our personal lives and enter our churches with miracle-working, supernatural power, we will never capture the world's attention. Why should we? Without His power working through us, we won't be any different than those who don't know the Savior. That's why we need radical men and women of God who will not bend, who will refuse to bow, who will not crumble under minor pressures. We need those who will not succumb to an ungodly world system, who want the fullness of God in their lives, and who long for a supernatural filling of the Spirit and God's anointing upon them more than anything else in this world, no matter what the cost.

When we read about the great revival of 1858, we need to notice that there were many contributing factors that set the stage for its manifestation. One element was a concerned group of Presbyterian churches across the land. The yearning for an awakening had come to hungry hearts, and out of that spirit came a special convention, held in early December 1857, in the city of Pittsburgh. The purpose was to pray for spiritual revival. Two hundred people attended the meeting. One brother under the Holy Spirit's leadership stood and said, "It appears to me that if we want to see God move, why don't all of us preach on the subject of revival on the first Sunday in January of 1858. And then, let us declare the first Thursday of 1858 a day of humiliation, prayer, and fasting?" With that encouragement—and its immediate implementation—the Spirit of God brought a grieving to their hearts. On the first Sunday of 1858, hundreds of pastors across America stood in their pulpits and preached to their congregations on the subject of Holy Spirit revival. Then, a few days later, on the first Thursday of that year, thousands of God's people across the nation took up the challenge, obeyed, and experienced a day of humiliation, prayer, and fasting for revival in their time.

What happened in 1858? One of the greatest moves of God this nation has ever seen. Over one million people acknowledged Jesus as their Savior out of a thirty million population in America. If we had a revival of similar proportions in this country today, in one year alone, we would see 8.5 million people come to faith in Jesus Christ.

WILL YOU PAY THE PRICE?

I cry before God for that kind of revival for us. As I fast and pray, God keeps telling me, "Ronnie, pay the price. Do what it takes. Get off your high-horse of ego-centered living, and live for Me alone. Get out there on the edge, Son. Don't worry what anyone else says about you. You might feel you're all alone sometimes, but I'm with you—closer even than a brother. Stay with me in humility, fasting, and fervent prayer. Know that I am God and that I will heal your land. But I will not do it until you and others come to me humbly, with contrite spirits, and with your whole hearts. Your job is to tell my people what I've spoken for generations. If you are faithful in telling them what I said—and if they truly love me—they'll do it. If they don't, they won't. You just keep on being my man. Revival will come to your heart and to your people."

I encourage everyone who fasts and prays—whether it is a one-day, two-day, week-long, or extended fast—to keep a fasting journal. This record will become two things in your life: a *spiritual guide* to help take you where you want to go with God during your fast, and an intensely *personal record* of what God is saying to you as you communicate intimately with Him *during* your fast. I consider my fasting journals to be pure gold—more valuable than any book in my library besides the Bible. They are filled with the words God has poured into my waiting heart. As I have reread my journals months later, I can see the issue of my human pride is one area where God continually worked with me. He was relentless. He would not let me go. He was the *hound of heaven*. And the more I saw my pride in contrast to His holiness, the more humbled I became in His presence.

OPENING MY HEART—AND MY JOURNALS

I'm not very *public* with my journaled thoughts, but it seems more than appropriate to share certain passages with you. Here are some of my reflections—taken at random—from both of my forty-day fasts as I wrote them in my journal:

> God's purpose in my fasting is to humble me so I can give all my energies to Him, so He can enlarge my boundaries and use me in a greater way for His service . . . I have had to go through the pain and endure the suffering to be used anywhere. God has given me a new power and authority.
>
> Lord, show me my pride as you see it in my life. Break me, God. Expose my sin to me. Empower me to repent of sin. Help me to seek Your face. Fill me with tears and a

heart for personal revival, church revival, nationwide revival, and global revival.

God, create within me an openness to You concerning
all things, freeing me from any personal or ministry bondage,
so I can receive all that Jesus wants to give and demonstrate
through me.

God, bring about a revival that will bring me humility,
brokenness, the seeking of God, confession and a repentance of sin that will fill me with tears and a heart for America
and the world.

O Lord, show me my pride as you see it. I have been so
blinded by it. Cleanse me of my pride. It is sin. It is a slap in
the face of God. I believe I need you, God, to come over me
with your power and your might. Unto you, Jesus, be the
glory and power. I give it all up to you and your power. I
pray today would be the day when God falls on me. Empower my will. I pray for a God-happening. Lord open my
heart to your Word. Thank you, O God, for your anointing. In Jesus Name.

Right now, God is on the brink of ushering in a great spiritual awakening across this land through this mighty gateway to
His supernatural power. When it comes in power, this awakening will be the manifested presence of God in the lives of His
people. It will cut through the clutter, it will demand we get
our spiritual houses in order, and it will happen only when we
keep our hearts and eyes focused on Jesus. This awakening will
be nothing more or less than a fresh, new awareness of the importance of obedience to God. It will transcend all man-made
barriers. It will come only when God's people humble themselves and pray, stand with God in His holy presence, and see

sins for what they are: conscious, willful alienation from almighty God. The immediacy of the hour calls us to act
now—not later. Revival will not come from the next election—
as important as it is to exercise our right to vote. It will not
come from playing church or maintaining the *status quo*. That
is a guaranteed formula for failure. Revival, and the spiritual
future of our nation, will be determined by the people of God
who will get down on their knees, pray, fast, and believe that
God is bigger than their circumstances, bigger than any election, bigger than the Democrats, bigger than the Republicans,
and much bigger than we are.

※ **God is on the brink of ushering in a great spiritual**
awakening across this land through this mighty gate-
way to His supernatural power.

There was once a page in the king's court. He did not have
many important responsibilities to carry forth until one day the
king called him into the throne room. The king handed the boy
a scroll, and on that parchment was written the following words:
"In the prison across town there is a man who is going to be
hanged today. I have decided to pardon him."

"Quickly," said the king, "take this message to the head jailer."

The little boy was excited about what he knew the king wanted
him to do. He ran through the town thinking over and over about
how grateful that prisoner would be, knowing he was now pardoned, and would not be hanged. As the boy passed a store, he
saw some clothes and thought, "You know, the prisoner will surely
need some new clothes for his new life." So he went into the
store and bought a splendid outfit for the one who would soon
be free. He ran a little bit longer, and then, suddenly, he saw a

place to eat, so he ran in and got some food for the convicted man because he knew the prisoner would be hungry. Then he started running with all of his strength toward the prison.

When he arrived, the young boy entered the jailer's office. With a smile on his face, the youngster took the scroll of pardon from the king and handed it to the head jailer. The boy said, "This is from the king himself. The man who was going to be hanged today is to be pardoned."

The jailer shook his head and began to cry. He said, "Oh, son, we executed that prisoner five minutes ago. He is dead. He is dead."

Tears welled up in the little boy's eyes as he walked out of the prison and headed back to the palace. As he shuffled toward the throne room, the guards could hear him mutter over and over and over again, "What is the king going to say? What is the king going to say? What is the king going to say?"

Our King, the Lord of Lords, Creator and Sustainer of all, King Jesus, is coming again. But before He appears, He wants to see a mighty awakening stirring in your life, in mine, and in the churches throughout this nation. If we don't choose to fulfill the spiritual challenges God has issued to us, we may one day walk away in grief, even as that little boy did. At that *kairotic* moment—that time of unconditioned reality—our last, fleeting, propitious moment before the judgment, you and I will know in our hearts that God wanted us to do something great through His power, but that we, somehow, were too preoccupied with other distractions to meet the challenge.

Then, on our way to stand before our God, it will dawn on us just exactly what we missed. As we approach the Judgment Seat of our Lord Jesus Christ, and come face to face with the King of Kings, the fear of God will overcome us as we realize it is now too late in the day to humble ourselves before the Lord, too late to fast and pray, too late to help others see God's gateway to supernatural power. As these thoughts slam into our hearts, we will find ourselves whispering those same words, *What is the King going to say? What is the King going to say? What is the King going to say?*

O Lord, do not rebuke me in your anger or discipline me in your wrath. Be merciful to me, Lord, for I am faint; O Lord, heal me, for my bones are in agony. My soul is in anguish. How long, O Lord, how long?

PSALM 6:1–3

I will praise you, O Lord, with all my heart; I will tell of all your wonders. I will be glad and rejoice in you; I will sing praise to your name, O Most High.

PSALM 9:1–2

CHAPTER THREE

Experiencing the Healing of God

IT WAS ONE OF THE LONELIEST MOMENTS of my life, sitting there silently, alone with my thoughts in the surgical clinic's waiting room. Watching CNN and reading a torn, dog-eared, month-old magazine seemed especially insignificant that morning. Perhaps as a kind of insulation for my fears, my mind began to work out the details of an important afternoon staff meeting, along with several other *important* events I had written into my schedule for the day. Then, something would shake me out of my planning, and every few minutes I'd glance at my watch and look toward the door that led to the surgical area.

Suddenly I was being swallowed by that cubicle, already feeling imprisoned by what I was about to hear. The words that Dr. Kendrick spoke still echo in the caverns of my mind: "Ronnie, your wife has cancer."

Finally, a nurse arrived. She took me to a small cubicle to wait for the surgeon's report on my wife's condition. As I sat there those few moments, I sensed this was not going to be a run-of-the-mill day. Still, perhaps out of denial, my mind had dismissed any thoughts that there would really be any kind of problem. I glanced up to see Dr. John Kendrick enter the room. By the look on his face and the somber tone of his voice, I knew something was terribly wrong. Suddenly I was being swallowed by that cubicle, already feeling imprisoned by what I was about to hear. The words that Dr. Kendrick spoke still echo in the caverns of my mind: "Ronnie, your wife has cancer."

I was used to seeing John wearing jeans and a T-shirt as he coached my older son's baseball team. I was accustomed to seeing my doctor friend at church where he greeted people with his usual warmth. It was only at this moment that it dawned on me that John was a physician who today had the painful task of bearing news that would change my family forever.

The moment he spoke those dreaded words, I asked him, "Have you told Jeana?"

He replied, "No, I wanted to talk to you first."

In 1984 Jeana had discovered a lump in her breast. We were concerned, of course, so she had a mammogram that was reviewed by a doctor in Texas. At that time we were told there was no reason for concern. Jeana continued to go in for yearly mammograms, and the response from the doctors was always the same: "We see no reason to be concerned at this time." The diagnosis was always, "Jeana has fibrocystic disease, not cancer." Then, in the fall of 1989, the lump changed. It became more defined. That's when I suggested Jeana see Dr. Kendrick, who counseled her to have a biopsy after the Christmas holidays. During that initial visit to Dr. Kendrick, he, too, said that he expected there would be no problem.

Now, today had arrived as uneventfully as any other Monday morning. Jeana didn't want me to go with her that day to the clinic. That way I could get Joshua and Nicholas ready for school. However, something inside me said I needed to go along with Jeana. I drove her to the clinic and then went home long enough to help the boys get ready for their day. I took them to the home of a neighbor who took them on to school. I then rushed back to the clinic to wait with Jeana for what I hoped would be just another normal procedure. After all, I was Ronnie Floyd. Mr. Organization Man. Had my day, week, month, and next couple of years penciled in right there in my daily planner. Ronnie Floyd: denominational leader, busy pastor—and a guy with lots of things to do today. I've only got a few hours to spare, thank you, so please, let's have a simple, insignificant two-hour disruption to our lives. Silly self-talk. But all my positive thinking and frenetic organizational needs would not change the results of the biopsy, the pathology report, and John's diagnosis.

ONLY THE BEST FOR JEANA

The reality of Jeana's cancer took Dr. Kendrick and me by complete surprise. How could a beautiful young woman only thirty-five years old, filled with energy and a love for life, have such a life-threatening disease? As he gave me the news of Jeana's breast cancer, my mind grasped for a plan of action that would end this nightmare. What should we do next? I told Dr. Kendrick that I wanted to get the best treatment in the world for Jeana, and that I thought we should perhaps take her to M. D. Anderson Hospital in Houston, Texas. My mind quickly filled with a hundred things we could do to take care of this issue today. After all, I was busy. I had not written the events of the morning into my calendar. I really didn't have time for this.

The nurse ushered me into the room where my wife was sitting. Jeana immediately noticed the look on my face, even though I was trying to hide my emotions. But could a man who'd been married fourteen wonderful years hide his feelings from the woman he loves? Jeana took one look at me and knew there was a problem. After unsuccessfully dodging her questions, I looked at her and said, "Jeana, you have cancer." The color drained from the face of my beautiful young wife. As we embraced each other, we both felt so helpless. The strong pastor and leader of a thriving church became so feeble, so knocked down, so quickly. John came back into the room and told us our options. He recommended that we see an oncologist, a cancer specialist, immediately. While Dr. John was honest with us as a physician, he was also comforting to us as a friend.

☀ **It was one of the most difficult requests I'd ever made of a pharmacist. I was asking for medicine for the woman I loved whose life was now truly in danger. How could it be? Not the Floyd family! Not my precious Jeana.**

The nurse helped me get Jeana in the car. Before we could go home, we had to fill a prescription for Jeana's pain as a result of the biopsy. It was one of the most difficult requests I'd ever made of a pharmacist. I was asking for medicine for the woman I loved whose life was now truly in danger. How could it be? Not the Floyd family! Not my precious Jeana.

We were numb with shock as we drove away from the pharmacy toward home. We felt helpless and alone. Gradually we began to talk. Should we tell the children right away? What should we tell them? Does our church need to know? How can we tell them? Since I was a visible leader in our area, this was going to be a challenge for me. We knew rumors would be rampant and magnified beyond reality.

Even though we felt alone, I can't say that we felt disconnected from God because within minutes the peace of God was with us. We knew God was up to something, so we promised Him we would not play games. We would be honest with everyone; we needed them now more than ever. All our family members lived in Texas, hundreds of miles away, so we especially needed our spiritual family to support us in prayer and love during this time when uncertainty was center stage and our imaginations were racing to the extreme.

CONNECTED TO GOD;
DISCONNECTED FROM THINGS

As we pulled into our driveway, I helped Jeana into the house. This would be the first of many times we would go through this procedure over the next several months. But little did I know at that moment how often it would be. After I gave Jeana her medication, she lay down on the sofa in our den. During those moments of fear and uncertainty, we prayed together for God's strength and wisdom. I remember saying, "Jeana, this just can't be. Is it possible that there's some mistake? We're too young for this." In disbelief, I cried out, "God, I'm thirty-four years old with nine- and six-year-old boys. They need their mother. What will I do if you take my sweet wife?" I needed Jeana. The boys needed her. We wanted to be a normal family again. Little did I know that things were not going to be anywhere near normal again for many months to come.

Even though I felt connected to God, I suddenly felt disconnected from many of the things and people around me. Problems, personal goals, and the office in-box, filled with other concerns that had previously been high on my list of priorities, no longer mattered much at all. Most of the plates I'd been balancing so carefully for so long just fell to the ground, shattered. All I wanted was for God to give my wife back to me.

Death to self is never without pain, but when God has done His work, and we have yielded and trusted, there is resurrection power and glory.

A. W. Tozer has written that the privilege of living in the glorious presence of God is open to every believer. Yet so many settle for remaining outside the Holy of Holies, content to "grow old and tired in the outer courts of the tabernacle." What prevents us from entering? It's not the character, nature, or actions of God, but the "veil of our fleshly, fallen nature," the self-worship that has never been crucified and repudiated. The sins of self are not something we do but rather something we are. We are afflicted with self-righteousness, self-pity, self-confidence, self-sufficiency, self-admiration, and self-love. Until the light of God is focused on these sins, we don't see them clearly. Strangely, some of the greatest demonstrations of these sins (egotism, self-promotion, exhibitionism) are tolerated in Christian leaders.

The opaque veil of self cannot be removed except in actual spiritual experience. Mere instruction will not achieve what the cross is meant to do. Yet removing the veil is painful, for it's woven deeply into our beings. Death to self is never without pain, but when God has done His work, and we have yielded and trusted, there is resurrection power and glory. [1]

Tozer was writing about Ronnie Floyd. Egotistical. Self-promoting. Covered with an opaque veil of self. How audacious of me to say in my heart, "Okay, God, you've got our attention with Jeana's cancer, now let's get her healed so I can get back to work. How could I have felt this way? What would it take to put me in the presence of God so that I could even *begin* to hear what the Father had to say to me?

OUR GOD REIGNS!

The day after we discovered Jeana's cancer, we went to see an oncologist. He painted a hopeful but honest picture of Jeana's condition. However, he told us that only through surgery could he accurately know her true prognosis. Exactly one week after learning of the cancer, we traveled to Houston to visit M. D. Anderson Hospital. I made arrangements for us to stay in a special room in a lovely hotel nearby. But in spite of the wonderful accommodations, the beautiful grounds, the art on the walls, the courteous staff, and the impeccable room service, that night was the longest night of my life.

The next morning my parents arrived at our hotel to take us to the hospital. On the way, I stopped to buy a tape of Christian music for my mother. We put it in the cassette player and let its words of comfort blanket our heavy hearts. As we approached the large medical center, a place where I'd visited the sick and the dying often as a pastor, I found myself gasping for air. Quietness filled my parents' Suburban as the next song on the new tape began to play, and immediately my mind and heart were encouraged with the lyrics of "Our God Reigns." My fears subsided. I could suddenly breathe. God had answered my prayer. He was with us. *He was with me.*

SHE REALLY HAS CANCER

The lobby of a cancer hospital is like no other. People of all ages sit in wheelchairs while others shuffle silently from one part of the room to the other, dragging their IV bottles alongside. Many are without hair; most are without hope. There is no laughter. Pain penetrates every crevice of the room. But the worst pain is not physical; it's a fear of the unknown. The breast surgeon met with us and confirmed Jeana's condition. He answered our questions and talked about the horrifying chemotherapy that loomed before us. The physician assured us that he would be in contact with Dr. Kendrick. He asked me to call him from the airport, at which time he would be able to tell us the grade of Jeana's cancer. This report would determine her future treatment.

While waiting to board our flight home, I called the doctor. He informed me that Jeana had what is called "nuclear grade-one cancer." In the grading of cancer cells, this meant her cells were angry and aggressive. Jeana cried all the way home. Reality had slapped us both hard in the face. Jeana had cancer. My spirit choked as I said the words to myself: *My Jeana has cancer. Jeana really does have cancer.* Tough Ronnie Floyd tried hard to comfort his cancer-stricken wife, when he needed a special comfort all his own.

☀ I must hear from you by surgery tomorrow or else, Lord, there will be no faith. I commit, due to feeling inspired, to pray and fast until after surgery.

And I knew exactly what I needed. I needed desperately to reconnect with God. This physical interruption in my highly structured life forced me to evaluate my cherished priorities. Suddenly, all those staff meetings, while important, were not as critical as I once thought they were. How Sunday's music would sound, and how many people would show up to hear me preach—all these once-paramount thoughts in my mind—were no longer my focus of attention. Instead, I found myself moving toward God. I was desperate for Him, desperate for His loving arms, desperate for Him to move supernaturally in Jeana's situation.

On Wednesday morning, nine days after the initial shock, I got up early and shared the following with God in my prayer journal: "Faith comes by hearing and hearing by the Word. We need a word today about Jeana's health. I must hear from You by surgery tomorrow or else, Lord, there will be no faith. I commit, due to feeling inspired, to pray and fast until after surgery." So I fasted and prayed—prayed and fasted. As I moved into God's presence in a vibrant, new way, I sensed He was honoring my fasting as I was connecting with Him in prayer. He has never spoken more clearly to me than He did that morning from the passage in Isaiah 43:1–3 (NASB):

> Do not fear, for I have redeemed you; I have called you by name; you are Mine! When you pass through the waters, I will be with you; And through the rivers, they will not overflow you. When you walk through the fire, you will not be scorched, Nor will the flame burn you. For I am the LORD your God, the Holy One of Israel, your Savior.

LEARNING ABOUT PERSONAL SACRIFICE

I had what I needed to be filled with faith. God had spoken to me in my desperation to reconnect with Him. Subsequent to her major surgery, Jeana underwent two minor surgeries to prepare her for the treatment to follow. She went through six weeks of radiation. Then she received more than six months of strong chemotherapy. During these months I watched her physical countenance change. Twice she lost all her hair. The Lord used this and the urgency of the hour to keep me before Him in fasting and prayer one day each week. I now know with certainty that God honored my act of desperation to reestablish a relationship with Him by submitting my whole heart to this time-tested biblical principle.

Most people know very little about personal sacrifice. Up to that point, I was among them. Personal sacrifice is when a person accepts the call of God, even when painful, to do what it takes to reconnect with our heavenly Father. During these difficult days God gave me a clear message that said, "Ronnie Floyd, the only way you are going to know My presence in your life is through the sacrifice and discipline of fasting and prayer. I'm asking you to give up the temporary convenience of food for a greater, more lasting spiritual goal. Your experience in My intimate presence will make you strong. You will see more clearly than you've ever seen before. You will learn to know that the same God who spoke to Moses, Isaiah, and Jeremiah is now speaking to you. I know you wonder why Jeana has cancer. Trust Me, Ronnie. I have brought you to this point so that I may use you as My servant in ways you cannot even now imagine."

Months later, my wife was asked by a reporter, "Jeana, where do you go from here?"

☀ "My job is simply to trust God daily, just as everyone else must do. None of us knows what tomorrow will bring."

She answered, "Well, we've had diagnosis, surgery, radiation, chemotherapy, and I don't know what to call this phase yet. It's just a new phase of the disease. It's a new step of faith and trust. I guess you have to come to the point where you realize that none of us has a guarantee of tomorrow. Simply because I have the knowledge that the disease could recur, I don't have to live in fear. My job is simply to trust God daily, just as everyone else must do. None of us knows what tomorrow will bring.

"Many times I claimed Philippians 4:6–7, 'Do not be anxious about anything, but in everything (even cancer and chemotherapy), by prayer and petition, with thanksgiving, present your requests to God. And the peace of God, which transcends all understanding (given to you by His grace—it really *does* transcend all understanding), will guard your hearts and minds in

Christ Jesus' (parentheses mine). I needed my heart and my mind to be guarded. I needed peace of mind, and I needed peace of heart. God was faithful, and He gave me just that."

PRAISE GOD . . . CANCER FREE

Jeana has now been free from cancer for more than six years. Today she has a growing ministry with cancer victims and survivors and their families within and beyond the church. God has used this ministry, the Cancer Network of Northwest Arkansas, in dynamic ways to minister to people, even bringing many of them to personal faith in Jesus Christ. Until we went through the pain of cancer in our own family, we simply were not aware of the magnitude of the fear and suffering in the hearts of so many.

I have told you this story is some detail for one reason: God moved in our lives when I allowed Him to touch me as He had never touched me before. Yes, Jeana was healed, but not everyone will be healed of every disease simply because he or she fasts and prays. I am confident, however, that as we pray and fast for the healing of our bodies, our prayers will be answered according to God's will and timing. Our only real prayer can be "Father, Your will be done." But looking beyond physical healing, God also wants to heal us from inappropriately defending ourselves and what may be ungodly actions, especially when they are indefensible. He wants to heal us from defeatist attitudes that are harmful to us and others. He wants to heal us when we don't choose to connect with Christ, when we blindly cast our lots with a church or religious institution where we enjoy the luxury of a business-as-usual environment, leaving little room for God to move us to the next level of relationship with Him. God wants to heal us from believing our own press releases—that somehow we have the inherent skills, training, and enough of a loyal following to do everything and anything in our own power. He wants to heal us spiritually, to draw us closer to Him, to keep us on solid ground, and to protect us from the influence of ideas that will push us off-center and away from the Father. He also wants to heal us emotionally, so that we no longer live the half-life of co-dependence, feeling we must meet the needs of others at any cost, and thinking less of ourselves than God thinks of us. He wants to do all this—and more—in our lives through the biblical discipline of prayer and fasting.

※ The self-denial and freedom of fasting and prayer provide a gateway for the supernatural power of God to come into our lives and minds, and advance the process of true freedom in Christ.

FASTING: MIRROR OF OUR DEVOTION

Fasting grows in value only as the discipline of fasting and prayer mirrors our devotion to God. Randy Sprinkle, who directs prayer strategy for the Southern Baptist Foreign Mission Board, reminds us that our culture conditions us to obey our every desire, which results in powerless bondage. But as Christians, God conditions us to obey His every desire, which leads us to freedom. Randy is right. That freedom releases God's Holy Spirit through us.

The self-denial and freedom of fasting and prayer provide a gateway for the supernatural power of God to come into our lives and minds, advancing the process of true freedom in Christ. After having completed short fasts and forty-day fasts, I honestly feel this enormous, almost indescribable freedom cannot be fully grasped in any other way. It is fervent prayer and fasting that reaches into the heart of God, motivates us to adjust to what God is doing, moves heaven to action, and changes what we see and do on earth.

As a pastor, I had become a reflection of my own denominational culture. Many in my denomination define success in relationship to how many people are baptized, how many buildings are constructed, and how large the budget becomes over the years. I have made the decision that I'll no longer worship the unholy trinity of baptisms, buildings, and budgets. That is *not* what being a follower of Jesus is all about. It's certainly not what a relationship with God is all about. I speak from my own experience, knowing God has brought a revival to this preacher's heart, and that neither I nor my ministry will ever be the same. That's because my primary inquiry no longer is, "What are You going to do for me during the next twenty-four hours, God?" but, "Almighty Lord, in humility, obedience, and surrender to You, how can Your purposes and desires be fulfilled in my life today?" God wants men and women of character, who are willing to pay the heavy price to experience His power, who come to Him not knowing the answers, and who approach His presence with the anticipation of being healed in body, soul, and spirit. But none of this will come about through a casual, walk-in-the-park relationship with God. It *will* come through trials, pain, and attacks by the enemy. The more intimate we are with God, the more it's going to rain on our earthly parade. We will come face to face with people, events, and challenges we never imagined. But because we have entered the gateway to God's supernatural power, we will also be equipped to do the work God has now given us to do.

WHAT DOES YOUR GARDEN GROW?

A Christian young man wanted to become established as a fruit grower, so he invested all his savings in a peach orchard. That year the trees gave promise of a bountiful crop. Then came a killing frost. In a matter of hours everything he had worked for was ruined. Embittered, he quit going to church. Finally his minister visited him to learn the reason for his absence.

The young fellow said to the pastor, "I'm not coming to church anymore. How can I worship a God who cares for me so little that He would let the frost destroy my peaches?"

The wise pastor thought for a few moments and then replied kindly, "Son, the Lord loves *you* more than your crop. He knows that while fruit does better without chilling winds, it's impossible to produce Christian character without the frosts of trial. God's primary concern is to develop strong men, not lovely peaches."

Byron Paulus of Life Action Ministries has written, "One thing that has gripped me . . . is the need for a renewed sense of urgency and fervency—the kind that welled up from deep within the hearts of men like Jeremiah and John the Baptist." Paulus continues, "A few weeks ago, the father of a friend of mine suffered a heart attack and was rushed to the hospital, where they tried unsuccessfully to resuscitate him. When the doctor gave the waiting family the news that he was gone, the grief-stricken widow began to scream hysterically. She could be heard throughout the entire hospital. At that moment, nothing else in the whole world mattered to her so much as the enormous loss she had just sustained—the loss of her husband's presence.

"When I heard that story, my mind went to the Book of Joel, where the prophet was advised of the impending Day of the Lord and the dreadful judgment that was to accompany it. Then he described in urgent, intense tones the appropriate response: "Awake! Weep! Howl! Lament! Fast! Call a solemn assembly. Cry unto the Lord. Blow the trumpet. Sound an alarm! Turn ye even to Me with all your heart, and with fasting, and with weeping, and with mourning: and rend your heart. Gather the people . . . assemble the elders, gather the children, and those that suck the breasts: let the bridegroom go forth of his chamber, and the bride out of her closet. Let the priests, the minister of the Lord, weep between the porch and the altar, and let them say, Spare Thy people, O Lord...!"[2]

✳ **When will we come to that time in our lives when God causes us to crave the nourishment of a spiritual feast *in His presence* more than bellying up to an earthly smorgasbord?**

That is urgency. That is falling down humbly before God. That is being aware of self and recognizing how hideous it appears when placed alongside the holiness of God. But where is that cry for inner healing in our churches—and in our world—today? Where are the sackcloth and ashes, symbols that show we have missed the mark, and that we need a holy God to set us right? When will we come to that time in our lives when God causes us to crave the nourishment of a spiritual feast *in His presence* more than bellying up to an earthly smorgasbord? For many, that time has already come. As of now, we have not seen the all-consuming fires of revival sweep across our own hearts and across our land. Still, in certain areas in America, a crackling of that fire is beginning to spread, even as it is becoming a wildfire in many parts of the world.

DON'T MISS THE JOY

Don Whitney gives us a good word when he reminds us that fasting does not force God's hand, but we cannot ignore Jesus' clear promise that God will bless a biblical fast (Matthew 6:17–18). If you have fasting phobia, it's important that you begin by confessing and repenting of your fear. God will hear your prayer and will prepare your heart to respond specifically to His call. *Be willing to fast as the Holy Spirit directs.* Often God will prompt you by a specific need—or needs—in your life that demands extraordinary prayer. There is no set length of time for a fast. Again, it is your obligation to follow the Spirit's leading rather than falling into legalism or taking someone else's experience as something to copy as your own. Seek medical advice if you have a physical condition that fasting will affect or if you feel God is leading you to an extended fast. If it's your first fast, start with the denial of only a meal or two. Withdraw during these periods of time to be alone with God. Let Him speak to you from His Word. But don't miss out on the unique experience with God that fasting and prayer can bring to your spiritual life. Don't miss the joy.

Throughout history, those who have allowed God to move with supernatural healing power in their lives have testified to the necessity of fasting in their lives. John Wesley instructed his followers to fast twice each week, and would not ordain a man to the Methodist ministry if he didn't do so. Others who recognized the importance of fasting as their spiritual worship and discipline include Martin Luther, John Calvin, John Knox, Matthew Henry, Charles Finney, Andrew Murray, and D. Martin Lloyd-Jones. And for what purpose? To be so healed from the sin of self-worship, to be so conformed to the image of Christ through their meeting God that they would become fit to make disciples. They knew their preaching had to emphasize the death of Jesus for sin, and the need for a sinner's repentance that would lead to forgiveness. The basic theology was there. But evidently only when they made the choice to access God's supernatural power through fasting and fervent prayer did the fire from heaven descend on their spirits and give them the ministry they came to enjoy.

Author John Stott once said that it comes more naturally to us to shout the gospel at people from a distance than to involve ourselves deeply in their lives, to think ourselves into their culture and their problems, and to feel with them in their pain. So, how do we learn to know the pain of others? Another question will answer that one: How do we come to know the pain of our spouses, our children, and our friends? Is it not by entering deeply into their lives? By listening? By paying attention to their needs? By caring enough to hold their hands when the tough times are descending on them like a flood? Is it not by entering the gateway to God's supernatural power to learn the discipline of fasting and prayer so we can know God's heart, and develop His sensitivity to those in need?

As I finish this chapter, I notice that my Bible has fallen open to a passage of Scripture that describes my deep thirst for the God of my salvation:

> As the deer pants for streams of water, so my soul pants for you, O God. My soul thirsts for God, for the living God. When can I go and meet with God? My tears have been my food day and night, while men say to me all day long, "Where is your God?" These things I remember as I pour out my soul: how I used to go with the multitude, leading the procession to the house of God, with shouts of joy and thanksgiving among the festive throng. Why are you downcast, O my soul? Why so

disturbed within me? Put your hope in God, for I will yet praise him, my Savior and my God. (Psalm 42:1–6)

There is a deep rejoicing in the heart of prayer. It is a rejoicing heart that says God will give you the answer to anything that may come your way. The prayerful heart is a confident heart, a thankful heart, an amazed heart. It is a God-filled heart that gives us the courage to look at our own small trials from God's point of view, even as we see, with greater vision and compassion, the needs of a world that doesn't yet know the Savior. In Jesus there is full joy—a joy that reminds us we have been healed, and that the Great Physician still makes house calls. He's ready, willing, and able to continue doing His healing work in our troubled hearts— hearts that have been changed forever because of our desire to be obedient to the Father's will.

They grumbled in their tents and did not obey the Lord.

PSALM 106:25

I will always obey your law, for ever and ever. I will walk about in freedom, for I have sought out your precepts. I will speak of your statutes before kings and will not be put to shame. . . .

PSALM 119:44–46

Chapter Four
Living in Obedience to God

SIR LEONARD WOOD was once invited to visit the king of France. It was such a pleasant experience for the king that he invited his honored guest to return and immediately set a time for dinner at a later date. When the day finally arrived, Sir Leonard returned to the palace. The king, meeting him in one of the great halls, said, "Why, Sir Leonard, what a surprise. I did not expect to see you. How is it that you are here today?"

"Did not your majesty invite me to dine with you?" asked the astonished guest, fearing he may not have come at the appointed time.

"Yes, that is correct," replied the king, "but you didn't answer my invitation."

Sir Leonard answered, "But your majesty, a king's invitation doesn't need to be answered, it must simply be obeyed."

Obedience is not a natural phenomenon for most of us. As children, we struggled to obey, terrorizing our parents with the most perplexing and unnerving questions we could possibly ask, and asking them nonstop: "Why do I have to do that, Mommy?" "Why can't I do that, Daddy?" As students, it was not much better, since we usually felt we'd probably be a lot better off if the administration would allow *us* to make the rules. And as adults, I have a sense we've not made a whole lot of progress in the obedience department.

LIKE A GOOD PILOT

"A good pilot does what it takes to get his passengers home," writes Max Lucado. "I saw a good example of this while flying somewhere over Missouri. The flight attendant told us to take our seats because of impending turbulence. It was a rowdy flight, and the folks weren't quick to respond; so she warned us again. 'The flight is about to get bumpy. For your own safety, take your seats.'

"Most did, but a few didn't, so she changed her tone, 'Ladies and gentlemen, for your own good, take your seats.'

> ※ **Just as experienced pilots do what it takes to get their passengers home safely, so it is with God.**

"I thought everyone was seated, but apparently I was wrong, for the next voice we heard was that of the pilot. 'This is Captain Brown,' he advised. 'People have gotten hurt by going to the bathroom instead of staying in their seats. Let's be very clear about our responsibilities. My job is to get you through the storm. Your job is to do what I say. Now sit down and buckle up!'

"About that time the lavatory door opened, and a red-faced fellow with a sheepish grin exited and took his seat.

"Was the pilot wrong in what he did? Was the pilot being insensitive or unthoughtful? No, just the opposite. He would rather the man be safe and embarrassed than uninformed and hurt."[1]

Just as experienced pilots do what it takes to get their passengers home safely, so it is with God. He looks into the empty, cavernous depths of our hearts and knows our deepest thoughts, even when we are not always fully aware of our inner world, and He knows what we need to do. Our heavenly Father knows, in this world of high decibel noise and permanent distraction, we will often fail to hear his voice. But He knows what we must do. When we think we need another class in self-improvement or a fresh prodding of our human potential, God simply asks us to obey His voice. When we're busy reviewing the blueprints to build our self-contained lives, hoping *this* will provide for our better future, God says, "Child, obey Me. I have better plans for you." When we think we finally have our lives under control because of our enormous wit and will, God tugs at our hearts, opens the pages of His Word, and asks us to read the gentle demands He's made on His children over the ages:

> In everything that he undertook in the service of God's temple and in obedience to the law and the commands, he sought his God and worked wholeheartedly. And so he prospered. (2 Chronicles 31:21)

> For just as through the disobedience of the one man the many were made sinners, so also through the obedience of the one man the many will be made righteous. (Romans 5:19)

> And this is love: that we walk in obedience to his commands. As you have heard from the beginning, his command is that you walk in love. (2 John 1:6)

SEEING WITH NEW EYES

Obedience to the commands of God comes through physical solitude, exterior silence, and by entering His holy presence through the spiritual disciplines of fasting and prayer. This is not an esoteric experience where we escape to a desert, climb a lonely hilltop, or retreat to the quietness of our family room for study without purpose. Our objective has never been more focused: *It is giving up physical food with a specific spiritual goal in mind.*

It would be presumptuous to attempt to guess where you find yourself in your spiritual journey. That is neither my purpose nor my desire. But I do want to try to persuade you to look at your life with new eyes—through the eyes of one who now may be starting to see that God has more for you than you ever imagined. To come to that conclusion, you must make your own decision that there's more to life than news, weather, sports, and ordinary religion. There must be more to your life than taking the kids to soccer practice, washing dishes, meeting deadlines, devouring fast food on your way to another meeting while on your cell phone booking another meeting, and ending up so drained that you wonder if you'll have the strength or the guts to make it through another day. And the harsh beat goes on until you're beaten to the ground. Whispering through the noise, Jesus is saying, "My child, there is a better way. Come into my presence. I will give you rest. Trust me, and obey."

THE FAST I HAVE CHOSEN

Solitude, quiet, and being set apart from the distractions of this world are vital to hearing God speak. If possible, I hope you'll be able to read the following verses in a place where you will not be disturbed or interrupted. If you feel so inclined, ask God to use this portion of Scripture from Isaiah 58 to speak to your heart, give your life new direction, and to demonstrate to you the kinds of results you, too, can expect when you live in obedience to God through fasting and prayer.

> Solitude, quiet, and being set apart from the distractions of this world is vital to hearing God speak.

Is not this the kind of fasting I have chosen: to loose the chains of injustice and untie the cords of the yoke, to set the oppressed free and break every yoke? Is it not to share your food with the hungry and to provide the poor wanderer with shelter—when you see the naked, to clothe him, and not to turn away from your own flesh and blood? Then your light will break forth like the dawn, and your healing will quickly appear; then your righteousness will go before you, and the glory of the LORD will be your rear guard. Then you will call, and the LORD will answer; you will cry for help, and he will say: Here am I.

"If you do away with the yoke of oppression, with the pointing finger and malicious talk, and if you spend yourselves in behalf of the hungry and satisfy the needs of the oppressed, then your light will rise in the darkness, and your night will become like the noonday. The LORD will guide you always; he will satisfy your needs in a sun-scorched land and will strengthen your frame. You will be like a well-watered garden, like a spring whose waters never fail. Your people will rebuild the ancient ruins and will raise up the age-old foundations; you will be called Repairer of Broken Walls, Restorer of Streets with Dwellings.

If you keep your feet from breaking the Sabbath and from doing as you please on my holy day, if you call the Sabbath a delight and the LORD's holy day honorable, and if you honor it by not going your own way and not doing as you please or speaking idle words, then you will find your joy in the LORD, and I will cause you to ride on the heights of the land and to feast on the inheritance of your father Jacob." The mouth of the LORD has spoken.

WE CAN'T MAKE IT ON OUR OWN

There are times in life when it becomes obvious we need the help of another person. A stronger person. A wiser counselor. A friend who can provide us with a perspective we cannot gain from our most noble efforts. The good news is that we already have such a friend. Perhaps we are troubled with physical infirmities, the mental or emotional pain of a family that's falling apart, or a financial crisis that is looming and has us scared to death, leaving too much month after the money is gone. Whatever our circumstances, there are—or soon will be—times when we will either choose to travel the highway to God's supernatural power, or opt for the low road of confusion, conformity, and compromise. Isaiah has a word for us at this point in our restless, overbusy, overcommitted lives.

We must consider ourselves blessed that God, through His prophet Isaiah, has provided us with twenty-two promises (results) that we can expect to receive from engaging in the spiritual disciplines of fasting and prayer—inseparable twins designed by our heavenly Father to usher us quietly into His presence. I have seen each of these promises come true in my walk with God, and I'm confident they can also live in you, through you, and will be yours as you call on God to do His will in your life. I encourage you to read and reread the above passages and sort through the twenty-two results you can expect from your time with God in prayer and fasting. I will share my thoughts on seven of these promises.

When we fast and pray, God steps in and frees us from the perceived alienation with Him that has kept us immobilized, fearful, and disobedient for so long.

Promise #1: Freedom

When we pray and fast, God promises that He will liberate us. He will loose the chains of injustice. He declares that He'll untie the cords of the yoke and will give the oppressed their long-awaited freedom. He will set us free from the bondage of what others think, making us realize that any comparison we make with others is a guaranteed fast track to misery. When we fast and pray, God steps in and frees us from the perceived alienation with Him that has kept us immobilized, fearful, and disobedient for so long. Freedom means we don't have to go to God to keep confessing the same, tired old sins we've been confessing all our lives, because God will give us power to do as we ought.

We are all too much like the faithful deacon who, week after week, would pray fervently, "Oh Lord, in your mercy, I beg you to clean the spider webs out of my life."

A fellow deacon, after hearing this prayer for too many months, in desperation finally prayed a fervent prayer of his own: "Oh Lord, in your mercy, kill the spider."

There comes a time when we need to move on—in freedom. As we come humbly into the presence of God in fasting and prayer, we begin to see our bondage in stark relief. Our sins show up in neon. What we were confident was acceptable, personal goodness, and righteousness turns out to be, as the Bible tells us, little more than filthy rags. But that's it exactly! It's that bold awareness of our alienated human condition that compels us to cry out for the liberation of our spirits. Before long, we learn there is a way of escape from our self-imposed prison.

As you consider God's call to fasting—perhaps for the first time—you may choose to start slowly, fasting and praying for only one day. Perhaps you'll decide to fast and pray one day each week throughout the year where you declare that specific twenty-four hours as your time of obedience to be alone in the intimate presence of God. I would suggest you begin your fast at 6:00 P.M., writing down the things for which you believe God wants you to fast, remembering that fasting is abstaining from food *with a spiritual goal in mind.* As you do, God will give you grace, comfort, and a new direction in your Christian walk. In the end, you will be set free.

☀ **Some studies suggest that 95 percent of us feel oppressed in one area or another of our lives. Why? Because, in most cases, we have chosen to be oppressed.**

Promise #2: Oppressed No More

When we fast and pray, God promises to break every yoke of oppression that crushes us. What's it like to be oppressed? We feel so ground down we wonder if we'll ever rise again. We've done our best, but it apparently wasn't good enough for some, and we became a bull's-eye for their mounting fears, anxieties, and hostility. The dictionary says that oppression is "the burdensome, unjust exercise of authority or power." It's precisely that.

Some studies suggest that 95 percent of us feel oppressed in one area or another of our lives. Why? Because, in most cases, we have chosen to be oppressed. We'd still rather remain in our bondage, calling for room service to come to the prison cells of our mind, rather than reach around and throw open the bolt to the unlocked door! God is the One Who's opened that door for you and me. He's already picked the lock. It's when we choose to walk through that door in obedience to His will through fasting and prayer that we receive God's anointing and power. That's also when we finally see our own self-worship for what it really is—an unholy act of pretending we are God, and that we have the wherewithal to run our own lives.

But when we give up food for an established period of time, with a specific spiritual goal in mind, we realize we are standing in the holiness of God's presence. We begin to hear, perhaps for the first time, His generous promise that our yokes of fear and bondage *will* be broken, that we are no longer oppressed by other "authorities and powers," and that because He empowers us, we *will* be free. The oppression of our pasts will no longer afflict us. The oppression of a negative spirit that is destroying our lives—and impacting others—will be left at the foot of the cross. Our oppression from problems so staggering that we feel we will never find solutions will be history. This is the power—the supernatural power—we expect when we come in obedient faith to the feet of our Savior.

Promise #3: Learning to Share

When we fast and pray, God teaches us how to share with those who have physical and spiritual needs. "Is it not to share your food with the hungry and to provide the poor wanderer with shelter—when you see the naked, to clothe him, and not to turn away from your own flesh and blood?" (Isaiah 58:7) The Book of Proverbs complements this passage by reminding us that when we give to the poor, we lend to the Lord. It's hardly the Madison Avenue approach to personal success and advancement. Instead of asking God to breathe His vitality into our lives, we have been sold a bill of goods on which most of us have already taken delivery. Instead of sharing with the truly needy, we become experts at piling up toys for ourselves. We somehow felt the more things we could accumulate, the greater would be the panacea for our ills—at least that's what the promotion promised.

> ☀ **The child without a father gets caught up in a gang, and the die is cast for a life of misery and pain. Where is the sharing of the abundance of our heart? When will we begin to believe—and act on—what we *say* we believe?**

But the package was full of Dead Sea thinking. Like the Dead Sea itself, we take, take, and take some more, with little thought of giving to others. We take in sermons for ourselves, but seldom give them away to those who are confused about life, lost, and dying without a Savior. We fill our homes with still more *things*, but we seem to keep these material blessings for the exclusive use of John and Mary and the kids, we four and no more. So much around us is Dead Sea thinking. Our self-help books promise us fame and fortune but are seldom able to deliver. The sickening, afternoon TV talk "peep" programs show us how low we can go in television programming. Our self-congratulatory infomercials feature pitchmen who hit us up on late-night television with the promise of a be-all-to-end-all skin cream that will not only make us look fantastic, but can help us finally say good-bye to those ugly little wrinkles forever. We're prodded to buy the latest, greatest exercise machine so we will have rippling abs and steel-strong thighs—as if that's the main reason God created us. We are promised we can make big bucks in real estate with no money down, so we can join the ranks of those millionaires who allegedly now live on Easy Street because they saw the light and got in early on the deal. Meanwhile, the widow goes hungry. The child without a father gets caught up in a gang, and the die is cast for a life of misery and pain. Where is the sharing of the abundance of our hearts? When will we begin to believe—and act on—what we *say* we believe?

Fasting and prayer put the sham life into perspective. These spiritual disciplines force us to ask ourselves, *Is this all there is? Is*

70

there not something more to live for than living for self? When such a prayer reaches the heart of God, He will respond, "My child, if you would enjoy a life of true liberty, see My face in those who suffer, see the needs of struggling humanity here and abroad with My eyes, hear their cries with My ears, and you will be blessed. I will show you the way you should walk, but you must come to Me humbly, obediently, in prayer and fasting."

Promise #4: Our Light Shines

Through prayer and fasting, God takes our dim, half-light of tentative faith and increases its candlepower so our lights can break forth as the dawn. We cannot look directly into the rising sun without damaging our eyes. Yet that's the kind of brilliance God promises will light up our lives and, in that glow, bring light to those dimmed spirits who continue to live in darkness. But it even gets better: "Then your light will rise in the darkness, and your night will become like the noon-day." A noonday sun is even brighter than the sun at dawn—and God is still talking about us. He's making us a promise that this will happen to *our* lights when we come to Him in fasting and prayer. We are indebted to The Christophers for their insightful motto: "It is better to light one candle than to curse the darkness." For you and me, it may start with that one candle today, perhaps another candle tomorrow, until we see that God is illuminating our lives with a beam of light that shows us who we really are, and why we need a Savior. The darker the day, the brighter our lights will become when we fast and pray.

As I observe those who have fasted and prayed over an extended period of time, I can always see that the lights from the spirits of their inner persons glow more brilliantly than ever before. That's because there is something profound about death to self, and an awakening to who we are in Jesus Christ. *This* is what brings a glow that God alone can give to people when they fast and pray. It's what brought such a radiance to the face of Moses when, on the mountain with God, he came face to face with his Creator. When we fast and pray, we, too, will begin to experience the glow of God that only comes when we go one-on-one with Him.

✺ If God's people are going to engage in the spiritual disciplines of fasting and prayer, *leadership must come from the top*—from those of us whom God has called to be His men and women of influence in our churches, our homes, and in the corporate world.

Promise #5: Healing for Body, Soul, and Spirit

"And your healing will quickly appear." Healing. Becoming robust and healthy in body, soul, and spirit. This is what our world cries out for: "Please deliver me from the pain. I can't stand it any longer. Will there ever be relief for my hurting body and struggling soul?" That's why we buy more pills than any nation on earth, yet most of our sickness is in our thinking. We're told the majority of people in hospital beds have no clinical reason for being there. *And your healing will quickly appear.* Is the Bible a medical book? No, I don't believe so. But it does offer a divine prescription for what ails us, and it declares its truth in the context of fasting and prayer. Many of us are stuffing ourselves with too much of the wrong food, drinking too many diet sodas, and loading up on too much fat. We are ruining our bodies with cholesterol, caffeine, and chemicals, refusing to exercise, and ingesting so much unnecessary over-the-counter medications that our bodies don't have a chance to function as God intended. We have choked the life, power, and potential from what God has called our *temples.* Let's be honest. If God's people are going to engage in the spiritual disciplines of fasting and prayer, *leadership must come from the top*—from those of us whom God has called to be His men and women of influence in our churches, our homes, and in the corporate world.

Fasting and prayer contain this healing element. For many years I was afflicted with continual headaches related to stress and allergies. It was nothing to have a headache each morning that would stay with me the major part of the day. Nothing would touch it—not aspirin or any other medication. But since fasting has become integral to my spiritual worship, I have been delivered from these headaches and all my futile attempts at self-medication, taking something like six aspirin and only one or two sinus pills in the past two years.

Was it the fasting that gave me relief? Was it the elimination of poisons and toxins from my body that brought on my healing? I don't have any idea, and it doesn't really matter. I just know I feel like the blind man healed by Jesus who couldn't explain how it all happened, but was robust in his testimony when he said, "I was once blind, but now I see." I believe God healed me. I have no reason to think otherwise. Our bodies, when given the opportunity to walk in obedience to God, *can* be cleaned up and healed to be the immaculate, highly functional *temples* our heavenly Father designed them to be.

Promise #6: Protection from the Father

Have you ever observed a mother hen looking after her young? If she sees a hawk circling overhead, she instinctively gives a warning sound, and immediately the baby chicks come running to hide beneath her wings. When menacing storm clouds fill the sky with rolling thunder and jagged lightning, she quickly makes a noise that calls her brood to herself where they find protection from the elements. As night approaches and the shadows lengthen, she gives out yet another, quite different, call that gathers her young to rest.

When we come humbly into the presence of God in prayer and fasting, our Father promises us protection: "Then your righteousness will go before you, and the glory of the LORD will be your rear guard." Protection from the front, and protection from the rear. God literally has us covered. And for good reason. Satan remains on the loose, roaming about like a roaring lion, seeking whom he may devour. As fasting and prayer become integral parts of our lives, we find ourselves overwhelmed by God's care for us, especially as our lives continue to be sprinkled with everything from daily annoyances to outright fear.

My colleague and friend, Robert C. Larson, who is assisting me in the editing of this book, called today and told me it was as if the enemy has declared *open season* on the manuscript. Bob's computer went down for several days; his father-in-law was stricken with heart disease and passed away; his mother-in-law's gentle heart stopped beating early one morning, and only now survives with the aid of a pacemaker; intense sickness struck Bob and his family, keeping him away from his computer keyboard for days at a time; someone from out of the past descended on him with a vengeance, opening an old wound, and further diverting his attention from our work, and the list went on. He said it, not in anger or self-pity, but with the awareness of how God's protection is needed, just as that mother hen senses danger and brings her brood under her wing.

Fasting and prayer will keep the enemy at bay. They are our spiritual shields. If you find it somewhat difficult to agree with what I am saying, perhaps you have not yet put yourself in a position to experience God's supernatural power in your life—a power available to you right now. It's simply not possible to live in the presence of our Protector and not feel the touch of His gracious, comforting hand that keeps our souls at rest while the storms rage around us.

When we fast and pray, we can expect two things: One, we will enter spiritual warfare as never before. That's why we must be prepared with spiritual weapons. We are taking over enemy territory. Second, we can know with all confidence that we are protected by God in the front and at the rear. Our encouragement comes from those who have walked before us in the confidence of their God—people like the apostle John who wrote, "Greater is He, (the Lord Jesus Christ) who is in you than he who is in the world" (1 John 4:4, NASB, parenthesis mine). Satan is our enemy, but God's protection is near at hand.

Promise #7: Answered Prayer

As you pray and fast, you will call on God and He will answer you. Answered prayer is the quintessence of praying and fasting. If I were to share with you the five or six pages of the prayer journal I prepared prior to my first forty-day fast, and then walk you back through my journal since then, you would see one thing: *My prayers were answered.* There *is* something to the disciplines of prayer and fasting.

You ask, "Well, what *is* it, specifically?"

I don't know. I only know that when Ronnie W. Floyd humbled himself enough to remove food as his focus to make the commitment to working toward a spiritual goal, when he quit trying to run his own life, when he finally gave up his best-laid plans and sincerest human efforts, and when he deliberately turned his life over to God once and for all, his prayers were answered. That's all I can say. "I was blind, and now I see." My experience with God's answer to prayer then—and today, as I continue to fast and pray—has ushered me into a new spiritual environment where I am no longer surprised at *any* of God's blessings. If anything, I humbly *expect* my prayers to be answered by a generous, almighty God.

When we humble ourselves before the Father, and when God sees we are serious about giving Him our broken spirits, He begins to do things we have never seen before. It's empowering. It moves us to another level in our Christian life. It sensitizes us to the bruising, almost impossible needs of others at home and overseas as we suddenly find ourselves quietly praying for people, events, and situations with the knowledge that our prayers not only will be heard, but that the Father will answer them.

INSUFFICIENT IN OUR OWN WISDOM

One evening Henry was in his pharmacy when a young girl came to get some medicine for her sick mother. He hurriedly mixed some drugs, put them in a bottle, and gave it to her. She took it and ran off as fast as she could. But as he was putting the various vials back in place, he was horrified to see that he had used one containing a strong poison. He didn't know the girl, nor where she lived. Perhaps the mother was already taking the deadly prescription. A cold sweat broke out on his forehead. Then at his wits' end, he remembered a verse of Scripture that went something like "Call upon Me in the day of trouble and I will deliver you." He began praying for salvation as he asked God to help him.

Suddenly the young girl reentered the store in tears. "I ran so fast I fell and broke the bottle," she exclaimed in distress.

Greatly relieved, he gave her the correct medicine. That harrowing experience got Henry's attention, and it's reported that from that day forward, he lived for Christ and became a different man.

Coincidence? Luck? Or God's timing, and *answer to prayer*? Does the fervent prayer of a righteous person make any difference? It did to Henry, the young girl, and her mother. And this experience can also be yours. Abraham Lincoln once wrote, "I have been driven many times to my knees by the overwhelming conviction that I had nowhere else to go. My own wisdom, and that of all about me seemed insufficient for the day." Only when you and I arrive at that cross-roads and make the same decision as Mr. Lincoln will our hearts be ready to hear God's call to come to Him in humility and obedience.

Obedience: Doing something because it is the right thing to do.

Obedience: A discipline that sheds light on the hidden things of God.

Obedience: One step toward God that's worth more than years of studying the subject.

Obedience: When believers who hear the promises of God give equal heed to obeying the commands of God.

Obedience: The most effective prescription for spiritual health.

Obedience: An act of worship that removes pretense from our prayers.

William Booth, founder of The Salvation Army, is on record as saying, "Go and get sure about God, and then you will have no difficulty in obeying Him—only get a proper idea of God, and you will be frightened enough of disobeying so great, and powerful, and holy a Being. . . obedience is only another word for the active side of religion."

On July 20, 1976, the Viking I spacecraft touched down on the surface of Mars. Programmed to work until 1994, it pleased scientists by performing beautifully, sending back information whenever it was asked—that is, until November 19, 1982. On that day, the Viking flight team at the Jet Propulsion Laboratory in Pasadena, California, radioed instructions to the spacecraft's computer, expecting an appropriate response. But no answer came. The *uplinked* message from earth was not acknowledged, and no *downlink* reply was ever given. Despite concentrated efforts by a team of experts, the spacecraft remains silent. No one knows whether it will ever respond to earth signals again.

As followers of Jesus, we have the assurance that our *uplink* prayer messages to God will never have that problem. We will never need to get on the phone and complain, "Heaven, we have a problem." If our hearts are right before the Father, the purity of our communication will never go unheeded, nor will He ever fail to respond to our deepest needs. This is the nature of God. He desires to know us, to work with us, to refine us, and to be pleased with who we are and what we do. In turn, He wants us to love Him, serve Him, live for Him, and to know Him with the greatest *intimacy* possible.

Answer me when I call to you, O my righteous God. Give me relief from my distress; be merciful to me and hear my prayer.

PSALM 4:1

The LORD is close to the brokenhearted and saves those who are crushed in spirit. A righteous man may have many troubles, but the LORD delivers him from them all. . . .

PSALM 34:18–19

CHAPTER FIVE

Enjoying Intimacy with God

I'LL CALL THEM Joe and Barbara Johnson. That's not their real names, but I want to protect their identity because of the challenges they continue to face even today. Here's their story.

Joe has had Multiple Sclerosis (MS) for more than twenty years. MS is a debilitating disease that slowly closes down the functions of once-healthy limbs, makes the strong weak, and brings the spirited to their knees. Joe was a strapping six-foot-three, handsome, 30-year-old with a CPA degree, and the comptroller for a major oil company when MS struck him down. One day he was running a corporation; the next day he was in a wheelchair on total disability.

Joe and Barbara have twin daughters, now grown with babies of their own. They have grown up watching their dad slowly deteriorate and their mother gently, lovingly, and consistently care for their dad, whose needs are ever-increasing. What I'm about to describe is what they've seen their mother do for their father week after week for most of their lives and how it created amazing intimacy between their parents.

Faithful Christians, Joe and Barbara attend church every Sunday morning, and then they often go out to lunch with some of their friends. In order to accomplish this routine, which sounds so simple to most of us, here's what Joe says has to happen every Sunday.

My wife is an incredible woman. Men not in my condition have no idea what it takes, both physically and emotionally, to be dressed and shaved every morning, to have someone brush your teeth, comb your hair, feed you, take you to the bathroom, wheel you out for a "walk" in the sun, and then wheel you back to the house where the whole process starts all over again. And she never complains or acts as if it's any trouble.

It's even more an act of love when Barbara takes me to church and out to lunch on Sunday. My girls have seen this routine many times, and they know how difficult it is. Before we leave the house, Barbara has to open the garage, back out the van, wheel me to the van, physically lift my six-foot-three hulk into the van, take the pedals off the wheelchair, load the chair into the van, close the garage, get back into the van, back it out, and drive us to the church building.

When we arrive at the church, Barbara has to do the whole thing in reverse, step by rigorous step. Go park the van, and wheel me into the church. About an hour later, we start all over again to go to a restaurant for lunch with some friends. Once again the whole process has to be done. All the time, she has this radiant, happy smile on her face, as if someone was doing her a great favor.

We sit down to have dinner, and she sits close by my side so she can feed me throughout the entire meal. She talks softly and kindly to me, and lets me eat at my own slow pace. When the meal is over, I know she's tired, but she's still smiling. She cheerfully pays the bill, pushes me out to the van, and the whole routine begins again.

Once we're home, she repeats the ritual one more time in reverse to get me back into the house, the van in the garage, and the garage door closed. Then she comes in and, invariably, says, "Honey, I really enjoyed today, didn't you?" That always leaves me speechless.

And if you think this whole rigamarole sounds overwhelming, just try to imagine what it was like when we also had toddler twins who had to be loaded into their carseats, lifted into high chairs, fed at the same time as I was, and chased around like other normal toddlers! I get worn out just thinking about what Barbara's had to do for me and the girls. She's the most beautiful woman in the world. God knew I couldn't make it without her.

INTIMACY: RARE AND SWEET

True intimacy is too precious for words. It is something God is just now teaching me in special, unique ways. I'm discovering it is an emptying of my soul in which normal images of life disappear, where words are no longer spoken, where the freedom of closeness with another reshapes our spirits as our entire beings latch on to the wonder—the unfathomable wonder—of the object of our love. For Joe Johnson, it was Barbara, his wife and helpmeet who loved him for who he was. She was a woman who did all she could for the man she cherished, without complaint and without regret.

Such a rare touch, this intimacy, especially when it manifests itself in the desert of pain where there is neither knowledge nor certainty of what may lie ahead. It is simply a moment to be in the presence of one's beloved. Intimacy. Pure love. Rare and sweet. It's the kind of relationship God wants us to enjoy with Him as He waits to infuse His mercy and love into our stressed and beleaguered spirits.

Intimacy. I am just now on the journey to discovering what it really means. I wonder where you are in your search. It's a serenity full of compassion and rest, giving us, finally, what we need most . . . to be held by the One who held the stars before He threw them into space, and Who touched the blind man and made him whole, just as our moments in His presence make us complete. Satisfied. Intimacy with God. It's one of the joys we can expect when we enter the gateway to God's supernatural power through fasting and prayer.

It demands we unclench our fists, check our unforgiving spirits at the door, pray that our fears and anxieties may be dispelled, and throw ourselves in humility and submission before His holy presence.

To achieve intimacy with God in our breakneck-speed world is not easy. Intimacy demands we make time to be in the company of the Object of our affection. It demands we bank the fires of our rebellious hearts and allow the Father to touch us, caress us, speak to us. It demands we unclench our fists, check our unforgiving spirits at the door, pray that our fears and anxieties may be dispelled, and throw ourselves in humility and submission before His holy presence. Discovering intimacy with God. Exploring intimacy with God. Enjoying intimacy with God . . . through fasting and prayer.

To know intimacy with the Father is to answer God's ancient question, even as it was put to Adam: "Where are you?" If we are honest we, too, must respond, "I was hiding." In our candor, we take the first step toward wholeness as we address our true condition. We are hiding from love, hiding from pain, hiding from our desperate fear of being known, and hiding from the God who loves us—who wants to clutch us to His bosom, never let us go, the One who wants to whisper a Father's word of comfort into our waiting ears. Intimacy.

To seek intimacy with God through fasting and prayer is to ask Him to break through the barriers of our bodies with our incessant demands for the creature comforts of food, entertainment at all costs, self-pleasures, and our insatiable pursuit of selfish desires. This kind of self-worship has never moved mountains of pain or created a legacy of love. But it has divided churches, killed relationships, put father against son, mother against daughter, nation against nation. Self-worship and intimacy are like oil and water: They do not—*cannot*—mix. When we are on intimate terms with God, we begin to see wounds healed and broken places mended, and we know Who to thank. Intimacy also demands that we ask God to break through the inner core of our minds, wills, and emotions, taking us into the virtually unseen and unknown inner sanctum—the deepest corridor of our beings where our spirits reside. To seek intimacy with the Father is to pray, "God, be everything through me that you already are in me. Put my life back in order. Help me know that without time in Your presence in fasting and prayer I have no other way to be drawn into the deepest recesses of Your love."

MORE THAN A FEELING

Intimacy with God is a lifestyle. If it is to do its work, it must change us from within and cause us to review and alter our behavior in the heat and torment of our days. Intimacy with God changed Moses on Sinai when he prepared to give God's Commandments to His people. Intimacy becomes a reality when you and I say, "That's me, Lord," to the question posed by the singer of the psalm:

"Who may ascend the hill of the LORD? Who may stand in his holy place? He who has clean hands and a pure heart, who does not lift up his soul to an idol or swear by what is false. He will receive blessing from the LORD and vindication from God his Savior" (Psalm 24:3–5). Intimacy with the Creator means baring our hearts to the Father, allowing Him to see if there is any wickedness in us. And how quickly the verdict will be read. But it will be read in love, with encouragement, and a prodding for us to return to our families, our work, our schools, and our churches as different people because we've been in the presence of God.

> What causes fights and quarrels among you? Don't they come from your desires that battle within you? You want something but don't get it. You kill and covet, but you cannot have what you want. You quarrel and fight. You do not have, because you do not ask God. When you ask, you do not receive, because you ask with wrong motives, that you may spend what you get on your pleasures. (James 4:1–3)

Intimacy with God begins with long periods of quiet listening, only later to become a conversation where we ask Him, in His timing, to repair the terrible breaches in our relationships, to bring healing to our tortured bodies, to remove our spiteful spirits, to help us speak words of kindness, and to learn to express unutterable joy for the flash of flame that now blazes in our hearts for having been in His presence.

Intimacy with God is founded on trust, faith, and love— the spiritual tonic we need in a distrustful age where these commodities are no longer in vogue.

The fear of intimacy (*into-me-see*) with those significant people in our lives leaves us lonely islands of discontent—sometimes quiet islands, but often islands with angry volcanoes that erupt and spew their hate over the unprotected spirits of the ones we say we love. But when we've ascended the mountain of the Lord, lived in His presence, been cut to the quick by His Word, and have been drawn to His holiness in fasting and prayer, we need to fear intimacy no more: We will want to know others, and we will also want to be known. Earthly intimacy will have a direct correlation to our intimacy with God, a closeness based on trust, faith, and love in Him. It's the spiritual tonic we need in a distrustful age where these commodities are no longer in vogue, where we remain terrified victims of wars and double-crossings in high places, no longer daring to place confidence in the leaders and institutions we once revered. In our own strength, vulnerability and openness to others will remain a formidable challenge; but when built on an intimacy with God, we will be given the strength to take the necessary risks to make intimacy with those we love a growing part of our lives.

AND GOD TOUCHED THEIR LIVES FOREVER

Those who fast and pray reflect that intimacy with God is the essence of their relationship with Him. Here are four examples of how God has moved in the lives of believers as they have stood on holy ground. They have given me permission to share their reflections, provided the emphasis is not on *them and what they did,* but rather on what God continues to do in their lives because they heard His call, obeyed His voice, and fasted and prayed. Duane Wilson tells how God called him to the new level of relationship with his heavenly Father:

Prayer and fasting started me on a journey of unbeliev-
able destinations. God opened a window of opportunity to
know Him as I've never known Him before. As I've become intimate with God through this experience, the Holy
Spirit has brought an overwhelming sense of unity and peace
to my life and to the life of my family. I prayed for several
months before I began to fast, diligent in my quiet time
with God—twenty-to-thirty minutes at a time—asking
Him whether or not this was something I should do. I recall so clearly the day God called me to take Him seriously,
and fully surrender my heart and my life to His control.

After the first day of my extended fast I had a tough
headache. My body had been loaded with toxins for so long
that physically I knew I would have to pay the price to have
them removed from my body. My headaches did not last
long. In fact, after a few days, I actually felt exhilarated. I
could see God as I'd never seen Him before. I could also see
my sins as if they were printed in raised relief. How could I
not have seen my selfish condition before? I loved God. I
thought I knew who I was. But I was living only a half-life.
Now, I was moving through that door to God's supernatural power, discovering real joy and true peace. One of the
things that was of concern to my wife, Bernice, was that I
had little interest in the mundane, but was fully focused on
the presence of God. For this time of fasting and prayer
God, and God alone, was my focus. I asked God to teach
me to love my colleagues at work, not just tolerate them, as
I'd done for so many years. My prayer journal was my guide.
I had a prayer list of seventeen items that related to my
work, family, and my deep desire to witness to my faith in
Christ. I drank 100 percent grape and apple juice with lots

of water, wondering, at first, if that would be enough nourishment for me. It was. I was tired at first, but before long, I was hardly even aware that I wasn't eating: My experience with God was my food, and His growing intimacy with me was my nourishment.

Within days, I was seeing everything and everyone around me with new eyes. I began to see people in depth. I could see their physical hurts and actually feel their spiritual struggles. I began to read God's Word with new understanding, asking myself, *Why didn't you see this before, Duane? It's been there all the time.* I prayed that God would not make me a stumbling block to others who needed to know His love in their lives. I was also afraid when I finished my fast that I might be proud of what I'd done. So my prayer was that God would remove any hint of pride, give me boldness and strength to share my faith in Christ, be more loving to those around me, enjoy a clarity of mind and spirit, and an abiding peace—all of which He gave me, in answer to my prayer.

I once thought a few minutes of quick Bible reading, a hasty prayer, and a "God bless you" to my family as I left for work was all it would take to keep me close to God. How wrong I was. I had to deny myself the most common thing of all—food—to put myself in readiness for the Father to speak to me. I can't speak for others, but that intimacy with my heavenly Father is what has turned my life around. I had been truly blind to the supernatural. Everything about me had been clouded by my pride, ego, and self-worship. But through my new experience with God, an awakening has come to my heart. I am more consciously aware of the needs of others, I no longer live anxiously, and when I put my head on my pillow at night, I experience true peace. But I do not want that awakening to stop with me. I want to be part of that greater revival and awakening that will soon sweep our nation and the world as believers begin to humble themselves in prayer and fasting.

SURPRISED BY JOY

I invite you to fast and pray for a spiritual attitude that will cause you to be surprised and overwhelmed by joy as you have your life-changing encounter with God. Most of us fill our day planners and our to-do lists with so many agenda items that we neither take nor make the time to listen to God. There is so little *God room,* so little time for what is truly important. Yes, we read the paper, check out the sports page, watch the evening news, but how important is all that, really? We need to work, pick up the kids from school, go to ball games, and attend concerts, but is that truly where we want our focus? Just that, and no more? Where is our desire for God? We tend to call on Him only when we feel we need Him, unaware that we will *always* need Him, at the beginning, in the middle, and at the end of any project or deliberation. And we need to come to Him in faith, not with high hopes or wishful thinking. That's not enough. It's faith that moves us into, and keeps us in an intimate relationship with God, and, once experienced, this intimacy is more real, more authentic than anything we could ask for or imagine. That was the experience with Christ that Doug Sarver was looking for when God led him to fasting and praying:

> God impressed upon me the thought "I have food you know nothing about." That's what got my attention. I knew all about the Bread of Life and the Living Water of God's

Spirit, but what was this food about which I was supposed to know nothing? I began with several shorter fasts that ushered me into God's presence, after which I worked up to a fourteen-day fast. At the end of that fast my wife, Karen, still did not fully understand what I was really doing. To put it bluntly, she thought I was crazy. It's too long a story to share here, but later our blessed God called us both to fast together, and we did it for His glory—a fast of forty days that was the most heart-changing experience of our lives.

But going back, I remember coming to the end of my first three-day fast, and how I was driving my car on a rainy day when it suddenly stuck me: *My fast is over.* I started to weep uncontrollably with the awareness that I had been in the holy presence of almighty God. Then, in tears, as I waited for the light to change, there was a crack of thunder, and the sky cleared as if it were a sign that God had heard the cry of my desperate heart. I'd been so involved for so long in doing good that I could no longer see my own sin.

That all changed dramatically when I threw myself before my God, praying that I would fall in love with my wife again, that I would become a friend of God, that my sins would be purged, that I would be freed from my quick anger toward my children, and that my faith would be renewed. Several verses from the third chapter of Colossians were spiritual nutrients for me during my fast:

"Set your minds on things above, not on earthly things. For you died, and your life is now hidden with Christ in God. When Christ, who is your life, appears, then you also will appear with him in glory. Put to death, therefore, whatever belongs to your earthly nature: sexual immorality, impurity, lust, evil desires and greed, which is idolatry.

Because of these, the wrath of God is coming. You used to walk in these ways, in the life you once lived. But now you must rid yourselves of all such things as these: anger, rage, malice, slander, and filthy language from your lips. Do not lie to each other, since you have taken off your old self with its practices and have put on the new self, which is being renewed in knowledge in the image of its Creator."

Whenever I share this supernatural experience with others, I'm always somewhat hesitant, because the purpose of fasting is to glorify God, not ourselves. Besides, fasting and prayer is just *one* work of God. That is not all there is. That's why it must not be seen as the latest "movement" to get us closer to God. It's not a movement. It's a humbling, one-on-one encounter with the living God.

When God calls you and me to share this intimacy with Him, then we will echo the words of the prophet Jeremiah, "This is what the LORD says: 'Stand at the crossroads and look; ask for the ancient paths, ask where the good way is, and walk in it, and you will find rest for your souls.'" For most Christians today, fasting and prayer is the path less taken. But when God calls us to walk that ancient path, we will find peace, comfort, and rest for our troubled souls.

※ It is often these unexpressed—and perhaps inexpress ible—thoughts that create the deepest intimacy with our Creator.

THE GOD WHO IS NEAR

For many Christians the only thing more troubling than attempting to talk to God in prayer is the fear of not coming before Him at all. Just as babies have a built-in desire to learn to talk, those who love God also have a built-in motivation to pray. Sometimes our prayers are only *sighs,* quiet aspirations to God when we don't have words to communicate what's on our hearts. It's often these unexpressed—and perhaps inexpressible—thoughts that create the deepest intimacy with our Creator. Fasting and prayer help us cultivate a dialog with the God who has already spoken to us; it's not a dreary exercise where we do our best to strike up a conversation with someone who must be coaxed and cajoled to become part of the discourse. It is communion of the highest order, a time when we literally enter the presence of God. This is what Chris Chapman experienced when fasting and prayer became an integral part of his walk with Jesus Christ:

> At first I felt left out. Was God not going to call me to fast and pray? Many of my friends were praying and fasting, and they were seeing tremendous results. And I have to admit that I was a bit angry with them for all God was doing in their lives while not much was happening in mine. But I had to know if this experience with God was really for me. In the end, I did feel that God was calling me to humble myself before Him in prayer and fasting. For the first few days of my fast I was terribly legalistic. Could I drink broth? What were my friends doing? What about vitamins? Could I exercise? I spent so much time wanting *to do it right,* that I was blunting the focus of my fast. It took me awhile to realize that comparing myself to others was a dead end.
>
> Slowly, I returned to the spiritual purpose of my fast: to come to know God in such intimacy that my life would be changed forever. I also prayed for my children, that their ear infections would be healed; that my sister, estranged

from her husband, would see healing in her family. I opened my prayer journal and looked down my list of desires, but most of all, I just wanted to know God in a way I'd never known Him before. It really is true: When we remove the physical, we then can prepare ourselves to grasp the spiritual. I honestly wonder if there really is any other way to know God in His fullness.

Now that my extended fast has ended, I have actually had even more spiritual challenges in my life. So I'd never want to give the impression that a fast is a quick fix, or a one-time encounter that puts you on a mountaintop forever. We all must come down from the mountain, but for those of us who've truly met Jesus there, our lives will never be the same. The best way I can describe my experience is that I was on holy ground. I know He's made me a new creation because I chose to walk that special path and enter the door to God's supernatural power.

Chris is learning that God does not need a tap on the shoulder or a wake-up call. God was there for him, even as He will always be there for you and for me, even as He was there on Mt. Carmel for Elijah when the prophet called down fire from heaven upon the blasphemous prophets of Baal. But what will you and I *be* when we enter His presence? Should we not approach our Father in solitude, silence, meditation, and with hearts receptive to what He has to give us? All the while, the most challenging aspect of our *personal retreat with God* will be to learn to close out the distracting clamor of our own agendas to listen to His voice. You and I will be tempted to tell God what *we* plan to accomplish during our times with Him, and there is an appropriate occasion for that. But that is not the primary reason to be still before the Father. We must cherish each special moment we pray with Him. We must savor the meaning of our fasts, and let our denials of food and outer disturbances lead us into His fellowship with such focus and clarity that the cares of the world are put aside. It was that focus and clarity that Tami Scoggins and her mother-in-law, Sara Scoggins experienced as they fasted together:

God not only called us to fast, but we sensed our God wanted the two of us to fast together. We are very close, and we wanted to be drawn even nearer to each other, even as we knew we needed to move closer to God. The amazing thing was that when we came to the end of our extended fast, we did not feel weak at all. If anything, we felt stronger physically, mentally, spiritually, and emotionally. We lived with Psalm 24 as our constant guide: "Who may ascend the hill of the LORD? Who may stand in his holy place?" We both wanted to climb that mountain to be with our God in a fresh, new way. And with God's help we did climb that mountain into His presence.

One of the most important things we learned was that we need to *choose* to come to God and experience his supernatural power. It is not an accident. It just doesn't happen because we're Christians. Sometimes we think, *Oh well, we can just go to church and we'll somehow automatically grow in our Christian faith.* But that doesn't always happen. When we obeyed God and began fasting and praying, He took us into an entirely different realm. At least that has been our experience, and we can only speak of what God has given us.

We had to be careful not to fast just because it was the *thing to do*, because it's never the *thing to do* if God doesn't call us to engage in this spiritual discipline. But we did hear that call. God confirmed our desires through His Word, and by what He was telling both of us—at the same time. We have found that fasting and praying has cleansed our hearts, renewed our spirits, made us more obedient to God's will, and has opened our eyes to see the world as it really is—lost and desperately in search of a Savior. Prayer and fasting has put us on holy ground.

SHARPEN THE AX

One day a young lumberjack challenged an older co-worker to a contest. Both wanted to see which man could fell the most trees in a single day. By sundown it was obvious the older lumberjack had won hands down. The younger fellow couldn't figure it out. He had chopped nonstop all day, while the older lumberjack had stopped every hour. When asked why he felt he had won the contest, the older man explained, "Every time I sat down, I sharpened my ax."

We can't cut down trees with dull axes, and we will never be the men and women God created us to be if our spirits are not honed to razor-edged sharpness by coming to the Father and enjoying the most intimate relationship of our lives. The counsel of the world is to stand firm where you are, don't take too many risks, get a strong grip on what's yours, and hang on for dear life. Be suspicious of everyone. After all, you really can't trust anyone, so you'd better trust yourself. Don't take any chances. Clench your fists, and no one will steal what you have in your hands. No thought for the inner life. No nurturing thoughts of peace or reaching out to others at their moments of physical or spiritual need.

The trouble with closed fists and closed hearts is that we set ourselves up for loneliness that could last a lifetime, never realizing we missed our greatest opportunity to know God, never knowing our clenched fists were the reason we failed to receive His gifts. However, if we go after our intended happiness directly, it will elude us. It will be like trying to catch a butterfly with our hands—a futile experience. Run after a butterfly, and the butterfly will win every time. But when we slow down, calm down, rest, and come into the presence of God through the joys of fasting and prayer, we will prepare our hearts to receive great gifts from His bountiful hand, just as when we no longer pursue them, the butterflies may come to rest on our shoulders. Yes, we will detach ourselves from *things*, but not for that end alone. We will distance ourselves from the distractions of life because we soon learn they are obstacles to our intimacy with Christ.

We began this chapter with Joe Johnson describing the woman he would never stop loving. Joe's wife, Barbara, was the love of his life. She was there for him *all the time*. Without her constantly at his side, he may have survived, but he would have been only half the man he has become. However, because of the almost inexpressible intimacy God infused into their two spirits, they became more *together* than they could ever have become alone and apart. That is what makes this such a memorable love story. You and I are like Joe. We are desperately in need of God, unable to get the wheels of our own lives rolling, incapable of taking care of ourselves. God is our food, our life, our sustenance, our very breath. But it's up to us to ask for His counsel and for His love. When we throw ourselves into His arms and become one with His love and mercy in the intimacy of fasting and prayer, we learn that what God has is ours, and that we can now have permission to leave our prisons of false-self to stand in silence before Him, aware of His holiness, the next secret.

You are not a God who takes pleasure in evil; with you the wicked cannot dwell. The arrogant cannot stand in your presence; you hate all who do wrong. You destroy those who tell lies; bloodthirsty and deceitful men the Lord abhors.

PSALM 5:4–6

My flesh trembles in fear of you; I stand in awe of your laws.

PSALM 119:120

CHAPTER SIX

Standing in Awe of the Holiness of God

GOD PROMISES to bless the efforts of those who stand in awe in His presence and serve Him with devotion and zeal. Jonathan Edwards, a faithful servant of God in colonial New England, was a shining example of a man with these godly qualities. Although his pulpit manner was not commanding, nor was he an extraordinary orator, many of his sermons had an overwhelming impact upon the people who heard him. What may be his most well-known message, "Sinners in the Hands of an Angry God," moved hundreds of his fellow countrymen to repentance from sin, turning them to personal faith in Jesus Christ. According to some historians, that one address helped fuel the spark that became the flame that gave the eighteenth century a nationwide revival and outpouring of God's power known as The Great Awakening.

QUIET STRENGTH

This may indeed have been true. From a human standpoint, it will always be difficult to credit such far-reaching spiritual results to a single discourse. Still, there's no question God used His servant at a time in history when a no-holds-barred message was needed to turn hearts toward God. But if Edwards' single sermon was indeed a catalyst for this great awakening, it was not because of his personal charisma. This preacher's approach to speaking was calm— a surprise, perhaps, to some, given the fame of his singularly most famous sermon. His hands did not flail the air chasing the devil from his hell, nor did he gaze wild-eyed toward the sky, calling down fire and brimstone from heaven. His power was not human. It was God at work in the heart of a servant who had been to the Holy of Holies. What many have not realized is this preacher of revival had never been *more prepared* by God to deliver his Spirit-filled sermon.

GIVE ME NEW ENGLAND

Those who were acquainted with the Reverend Edwards knew that prior to the delivery of his message he had not eaten a mouthful of food for three days, nor, during that time, had he closed his eyes in sleep. Instead of pouring nutrients into his body, he sated his hungry soul with the food of the Spirit; instead of giving in to sleep, he pursued communion with His God that was as deep and far-reaching as any time ever in God's presence. Over and over Edwards was heard to pray, "O Lord, give me New England! Lord, give me New England!" Lathered in sweat and tears, when Jonathan Edwards rose from his knees and made his way into the pulpit that historic Sunday, those who saw him were transfixed, saying later that he looked as though he had been gazing straight into the face of God. Three days of fasting and praying had prepared his heart to preach the sermon of his life.

> **Over and over he was heard to pray, "O Lord, give me New England! Lord, give me New England!"**

Even before he began to speak, said eyewitnesses, spiritual dread and the heaviness of a conviction of sin fell upon his audience. And then he spoke his message, "Sinners in the Hands of an Angry God." He held his sermon notes so close that the audience could not see his face. He preached and preached until the people in that crowded assembly were moved almost beyond control. It's said that one man jumped up and rushed down the aisle crying, "Mr. Edwards, have mercy!" Others clutched the backs of the pews for fear of falling into the fiery pit of hell itself. Most thought the day of judgment had dawned. And for some, undoubtedly it had. Everyone in that assembly found himself standing in awe of the holiness of God.

THE CHRISTIAN'S MANDATE

Entering God's presence through prayer and fasting prepares the way for us to catch a glimpse of God's holiness. Adrian Rogers says, "The church advances on its knees. Few things are talked about more in church than prayer, yet relatively few saints know and experience the marvels of intercession. The chief weapon against Satan is prayer. Satan has many strongholds, many bastions of strength in America today. To try to break them down with Madison Avenue techniques would be as worthless as trying to remove the Rock of Gibraltar by throwing snowballs at it. Satan sneers at our schemes, mocks our methods, laughs at our learning, but is paralyzed by our praying."

It is this awareness of what our strength *is*, and what it *is not*, that gives us our direction in the violent atmosphere of spiritual warfare in which we live. We cannot be salt and light and leaven to a world in despair by using tricks and methods that are at best ineffective. Questionable religious schemes always produce spurious results, the ecclesiastical equivalent of rearranging the chairs on the Titanic, hoping the singing of *Nearer My God to Thee* will somehow save the day. It never has and never will. To anesthetize the strongholds of the enemy is to come face to face with the holiness of God by entering His presence through fasting and praying with a repentant heart. As we do, we learn that God has no need for us, but that we have a desperate need for Him. His purity will be more than we can bear. His righteousness is so great that our feeble hearts will not be able to accommodate His glory. His sinlessness is so overwhelming that, in tears and with faces to the ground, we will be driven to see ourselves for who we really are—aliens from a holy God, distant from His uncompromising truth, suddenly discovering what we need most is to speak the words of the prophet Isaiah, admitting our own estrangement from our heavenly Father:

> Woe to me! . . . I am ruined! For I am a man of unclean lips, and I live among a people of unclean lips. . . . (Isaiah 6:5)

> Woe to those who are wise in their own eyes and clever in their own sight. (Isaiah 5:21)

> "Woe to the obstinate children," declares the LORD, "to those who carry out plans that are not mine, forming an alliance, but not by my Spirit, heaping sin upon sin." (Isaiah 30:1)

FILLED WITH THE SPIRIT; EMPOWERED BY THE SPIRIT

During my times of fasting and prayer, God invariably directs my heart to verses such as these. As I read, I become broken in His presence, see my obstinate heart, recognize that I am of unclean lips, continually worshiping at the altar of self. Again and again I have had to admit before God that I still often try to hide my cleverness under a cloak of ministerial privilege. What I need now is what Jesus himself experienced after He fasted and prayed for forty days while being tempted by Satan. He went up that desert mountain filled with the Spirit, but as Luke 4:14 reminds us, "Jesus returned to Galilee *in the power of the Spirit,* and news about him spread through the whole countryside" (italics mine). It is essential that the Spirit of God fill us, even as it filled our Savior. But our strength for a life of witness comes when we, like Jesus, live *in the power of the Spirit.* If the gospel does not empower us to a personal awakening, if it does not make us sorrowful for a nation without God, and if we are not moved to want to touch a world that does not name the name of Jesus, we have failed to capture what it means to have been in the holy presence of God.

It is essential that the Spirit of God fill us, even as it filled our Savior. Our strength for a life of witness comes when we, like Jesus, live *in the power of the Spirit.*

When working on the pages of my fasting journals, I felt the hand of God direct my pen as I wrote . . .

> Heavenly Father, break me, expose my sin to me, empower me to repent of my sin, help me to seek Your face. Fill me with tears and a heart for personal revival, church revival, nationwide revival, and global revival. God, endow me with the authority and power of Jesus Christ in everything I do. Help me know Your holiness, whatever the cost. I am willing to pay the price for being in Your presence. God, pour out Your Spirit in such a way that a mighty revival and an awakening to Your power break out among those who hear the message You have given me to share. God, give me a revival in my heart for those who don't know You, filling my mouth so much with Jesus that I will tell everyone I meet of my

Savior and of His love for them, and how You can bring hope and healing to their shattered lives. Lord, I ask in Your mercy, to create within me an openness to all things that are truly from You, holy God. Free me from any personal or ministry bondage so that I may receive all of You that You want to give me and demonstrate through me. God, show me your holiness. Dear God, show me Your holiness.

God did not fail to show me His holiness. He also honored the desires of my heart and changed my spirit forever.

INVENTORY OF THE HEART

I have kept the following verses and their poignant, embarrassing questions close at hand during my fasts as a reminder that, if I was going to be serious about knowing God's holiness, I would need to look at an entire landscape of issues. I share these with you with a heart that invites you to be quietly honest with yourself and honest with God as you reflect on your answers. This is an important exercise, because when you and I choose to enter the gateway to God's supernatural power and live in the presence of His holiness, we must become persuaded that every yes to these questions suggests there is a sin for us to confess. I have long lived with these heart-piercing Scriptures and provocative questions. Now I share them with you and join you in this personal inventory of the heart.

1. *In everything give thanks, for this is the will of God in Christ Jesus for you.* (1 Thessalonians 5:18, NKJV)
   Do we worry about anything? Have we forgotten to thank God for all things, the seemingly bad as well as the good? Do we neglect to give Him thanks for our breath, our health, and for life itself?

2. *Now to Him who is able to do exceedingly abundantly above all that we ask or think, according to the power that works in us.* (Ephesians 3:20, NKJV)
Do we shy away from attempting to do things in the name of our heavenly Father because we fear we are not talented enough? Do feelings of inferiority keep us from our desire to serve God? When we do accomplish something of merit, do we choose to give ourselves, rather than God, the glory?

3. *You shall receive power when the Holy Spirit has come upon you; and you shall be witnesses to Me in Jerusalem, and in all Judea and Samaria, and to the end of the earth.* (Acts 1:8, NKJV)
Have we been hesitant to thank God for the miracles He has performed in our lives? Have we believed it's good enough to live our Christianity in a casual manner, and that it's not all that important to share the good news of our deliverance with others?

4. *I say . . . to everyone who is among you, not to think of himself more highly than he ought to think. . . .* (Romans 12:3, NKJV)
Are we overly proud of our accomplishments, our talents, our families? Do we have difficulty putting the concerns of others first? Do we have a rebellious spirit at the thought that God may want to change us, and rearrange our thinking?

5. *Let all bitterness, wrath, anger, clamor, and evil speaking be put away from you, with all malice.* (Ephesians 4:31, NKJV)
Do we complain, find fault, argue? Do we nurse, and delight in, a critical spirit? Do we carry a grudge against believers of another group, denomination, or theological persuasion because they don't see the truth as we see it? Do we speak unkindly about people when they are not present? Do we find that we're often angry with ourselves? With others? With God?

6. *Do you not know that your body is the temple of the Holy Spirit who is in you, whom you have from God, and you are not your own?* (1 Corinthians 6:19, NKJV)

   Are we careless with our bodies? Do we defile our bodies with unholy sexual acts?

7. *Let no corrupt communication proceed out of your mouth. . . .* (Ephesians 4:29, NKJV)

   Do we use language that fails to edify others, tell off-color jokes or stories that demean another person's race, habits, or culture? Do we condone these comments when guests are in our home or when our colleagues share them with us at work?

8. *Do not . . . give place to the devil.* (Ephesians 4:26–27, NKJV)

   Do we close our eyes to the possibility that we may be a landing strip for Satan when we open our minds to him through ungodly practices, psychic predictions, occult literature, and violent, sex-driven, sexually-perverted movies and videos? Do we seek counsel for daily living from horoscopes in the paper, on television, or on the Internet rather than from God, our true and ultimate source for living? Do we let Satan use us to set up barriers that inhibit the cause of Christ in our churches and in our homes through criticism and gossip?

9. *Not slothful in business. . . .* (Romans 12:11, KJV)

   Are we chronically late in paying our debts, sometimes choosing not to pay them at all? Do we charge more on our credit cards than we can honestly afford to pay? Do we neglect to keep honest income tax records? Do we engage in shady business deals?

10. *Beloved . . . abstain from fleshly lusts which war against the soul.* (1 Peter 2:11, NKJV)

Are we guilty of a lustful eye toward the opposite sex? Do we fill our minds with sexually oriented TV programs, lewd movies, unsavory books and magazines? Their covers? Centerfolds? Especially when we sense no one is watching? Do we indulge in lustful activities that God's Word condemns, such as fornication, adultery, perversion?

11. *Bearing with one another, and forgiving one another, if any-one has a complaint against another; even as Christ forgave you, so you also must do.* (Colossians 3:13, NKJV)
Have we failed to forgive those who may have said or done something to hurt us? Have we written off certain people as not worthy of our friendship?

12. *Even so you also outwardly appear righteous to men, but inside you are full of hypocrisy and lawlessness.* (Matthew 23:28, NKJV)
Do we know in our hearts that we are often not what people see? Are we possibly hiding behind being active in our churches as a cover for our activities away from the Body of Christ? Are we mimicking the Christian faith for social status, acceptance in our church or our community? Are we real?

13. *Finally, brethren, whatever things are true, whatever things are noble, whatever things are just, whatever things are pure, whatever things are lovely, whatever things are of good report, if there is any virtue and if there is anything praiseworthy— meditate on these things.* (Philippians 4:8, NKJV)
Do we enjoy listening to conversation that hurts others? Do we pass it on? Do we believe rumors or partial truths, especially about an enemy or a competitor? Do we choose to spend little or no time each day allowing God to speak to us through His Word?

CHANGED LIVES OR NOTHING AT ALL

These are hard sayings and tough questions. At first, I hesitated to include these because they are so laser-like, so straight to the heart, brutal, and to the point. Then, the Spirit of God instructed me not to pull any punches. If we don't address these questions with honest hearts, the chances for personal renewal are virtually nil. We cannot play games with God and, at the same time, experience a spiritual awakening. Christianity in an unawakened America has already reached a level of diminishing returns. Richard Foster says, "People do not see anything to be converted to. They look around at these Christians telling them to agree to these little statements and say the enclosed prayer. They say, 'But you aren't any different from anybody else. So what am I supposed to be converted to?' We have to see changed lives."

Changed lives. *Results* from being in the holy presence of God. Changed attitudes, changed relationships, changed hearts. This is what can happen when we experience the supernatural power of God through fasting and prayer. When we repent of our willful desire to put distance between ourselves and God's holiness, He will change our attitudes toward our most cherished sins, and we will find ourselves in the center of a spiritual breakthrough. Only as we live in His presence will the power of the Holy Spirit enable us to change both our attitudes *and* our conduct. Instead of doing what our self-worshiping nature wants to do, we will choose to do what God wants us to do. When we experience God's holiness through fasting and prayer—giving up what is natural to attain a spiritual goal—we will never be the same. God will give us liberty. We will know the meaning of true worship. Our sinfulness, hopelessness, and insufficiency will come so clearly to the forefront that we, like the hearers of Jonathan Edwards' sermon—will know we are but one step from destruction. This is what can happen to us when we stand in awe of the holiness of God.

☀️ They say, "But you aren't any different from anybody else. So what am I supposed to be converted to?" We have to see changed lives.

GOD IS NOT SAFE!

In *The Chronicles of Narnia*, a series of allegories by C. S. Lewis, the author describes two girls, Susan and Lucy, getting ready to meet Aslan the lion, who represents Christ. Two talking animals, Mr. and Mrs. Beaver, prepare the children for the encounter.

"Ooh," said Susan, "I thought he was a man. Is he quite safe? I shall feel rather nervous about meeting a lion."

"That you will, dearie," said Mrs. Beaver. "And make no mistake, if there's anyone who can appear before Aslan without their knees knocking, they're either braver than most or else just silly."

"Then, isn't he safe?" said Lucy.

"Safe," said Mr. Beaver. "Don't you hear what Mrs. Beaver tells you? Who said anything about safe? Of course, he isn't safe, but he's good. He's the king, I tell you!"

NO LONGER ALIENS

The psalmist understood this awesome wonder when he wrote, "Taste and see that the Lord is good. . . ." and then urged God's saints to fear Him (Psalm 34:8–9). We need not cringe in terror, but we must live before Him with reverence and awe. Our holy God is not *safe*, but He is good. In fact, God is highly dangerous as long as we remain aliens from His grace. Our willful trespasses can no more exist in the presence of God than darkness can coexist with the light. To stand before God is to invite destruction, just as Moses knew he would have died had he looked into the face of God.

✺ **Holiness expresses itself with greatest integrity when our primary motive in life is the passionate desire to please God with our whole hearts.**

Then comes the comforting message of hope—that we are clean in our Father's sight, without spot or wrinkle, whole and healed. But this will not be a *cheap grace*. We are not allowed to take His holiness for granted. Nor are we to regard it as a theological concept to be studied and kept under lock and key. By definition, holiness means to be separated and set apart, which is its purpose for us in our daily lives. Holiness will always have more to do with our inward lives than our outward expressions. Holiness will express itself with greatest integrity when our primary motive in life is the passionate desire to please God with our whole hearts. Holiness also leads to humanness—not depraved humanity, but life to be lived as God intended, perfectly expressed in the life of our Savior. Secular humanists have perverted the concept of humanness. Rather than cherishing God's ideal for human life, they deify self and deny God. Only through Jesus Christ will we ever become truly human—the kind of people God designed us to be.

Without a regular encounter with God and his holiness, we will still default to a business-as-usual attitude toward God and life, just like the good ol' boy who came walking down the path from the Carolina mountains one day. He was all dressed up and carrying his Bible.

A friend saw him and asked, "Elias, what's happening? Where are you going all dressed up like that?"

Elias said, "I'm heading for New Orleans. I've been hearing that there's a lot of free-runnin' liquor and a lot of gamblin' and a whole lot of real good naughty shows."

His friend looked him over and said, "But Elias, why are you carrying your Bible under your arm?"

Elias answered, "Well, if it's as good as they say it is, I might just stay over until Sunday."

What Elias never learned was that when we spend time with God, we must change, even as we continue to function in the world of reality, touch real people, and make decisions about real problems. But because we've been with God, we will see people and events with God's eyes and with God's heart. This is where we are to live out the holiness God has given us, something that is neither outdated nor optional. Today, there are endless programs of evangelizing that stress everything but God's holiness. Most of our leaders are not valued for their holiness, but for their ability to draw a crowd, thrill a crowd, and hold a crowd, thanks to their communication skills or political clout. How far this is from entering God's gateway to supernatural power. J. I. Packer says, "Holiness is the very purpose of regeneration: that believers become Christlike. Nothing defeats Satan's purposes for Christians like a holy life, and nothing plays into his hands more than the failure to practice holiness. Holiness gives credibility to witness; lack of it negates the witness. True happiness comes only as a by-product of holiness."

HOLINESS IN ACTION

A missionary in India was once teaching the Bible to a group of Hindu ladies. Halfway through the lesson, one of the women got up and walked out. A short time later, she came back and listened more intently than ever.

At the close of the hour the leader inquired, "Why did you leave the meeting? Weren't you interested?"

"Oh yes," the Hindu lady replied. "I was so impressed with what you had to say about Christ that I went out to ask your carriage driver whether you really lived the way you talked. When he said you did, I hurried back so I wouldn't miss out on anything."

So my questions to you and to me are these:

> What would He find, should He come just now?
> A faded leaf or a fruitless bough;
>
> A servant sleeping, an idle plow;
> What would He find should He come just now?
> What would He find should He come tonight,
>
> Our garments soiled or a spotless white;
> Our lamps all burning or with no light;
> What would He find should He come tonight?

The privilege of living in the presence of God is open to every believer. Yet many of us settle for remaining outside that Holy of Holies, satisfied to grow weary and old in the outer courts of the tabernacle. What prevents us from entering this gateway to God's supernatural power? It's not the character, nature, or actions of God, but the darkened veil of our own self-worship, a self-life that has not been carried to the foot of the cross.

In the end, it's the small things that will make or break us. Everything we do counts, just as each stone in a beautiful mosaic counts *because each stone is vital to the life of the art.* A life lived wholly for God is also constructed of a myriad of small things. It is the little things of the moment, and not the great things of the age, that must captivate our lives. It's the kind, but little, words of faith, not the eloquent, heady lectures or overly organized sermons; it's the small acts of kindness and our personal witness to God's saving love, not the difficult-to-believe miracles or high-profile spiritual battles; it's the still waters of Siloam that provide healing for the sick and the dying, not the raging torrents that scream their fury, calling attention to themselves. It's always the small things that are the quiet symbols of a holy life.

THE GANGSTER SAID NO!

Several years ago a prominent underworld figure attended a large evangelistic crusade. Realizing that the cause of evil would be weakened if this man were converted, those conducting the meeting talked to him about a relationship with Christ. One night they urged him to open the door of his heart and allow the Savior to enter his life. The man supposedly embraced Christ as Lord, but as the months passed his lifestyle remained the same. When confronted with this inconsistency, the gangster said no one had told him that in saying yes to Jesus he would be turning his back on his former occupation. After all, he reasoned, there were Christian football players, Christian cowboys, Christian politicians— why not a Christian gangster? Only then did his Christian friends explain his need for repentance. Upon hearing this, the man turned away, wanting nothing to do with Jesus. The gangster was unwilling to pay the price. He could not see his way clear to edge toward the gateway that led into the presence of the living God.

The gangster said no. It's my prayer that you will say yes to God's invitation to know Him in such a way that your life will never be the same again. God wants to tell us His secrets—secrets we will never hear unless we enter His presence humbly, silently, with hearts free from the distractions of life. He wants to manifest Himself in our lives as He waits patiently for us to place our lives under His command and His influence, so that He may do for us *once* what He promises to do for us *forever*. We must not remain stuck in the turmoil of life and its cares or we may never know His power. We must not be so eager to ask our own questions that we cannot hear God's answers. Only as we stand in His holy presence will we hear one of the greatest desires of our Father's heart—a full, complete, and absolute surrender to Him in *every* area of our lives . . . an all-too-forgotten secret.

Awake, O Lord! Why do you sleep? Rouse yourself! Do not reject us forever. Why do you hide your face and forget our misery and oppression?

PSALM 44:23–24

Praise the LORD, all you servants of the LORD who minister by night in the house of the LORD. Lift up your hands in the sanctuary and praise the LORD.

PSALM 134:1–2

CHAPTER SEVEN

Surrendering Fully to God

HE WAS GOD'S MAN sent in God's time. He had only one commitment: to see men and women come to faith in Jesus Christ and to give their lives in full surrender to their heavenly Father. A prophet to his own generation, he despised the devil, hated sin, and declared that "booze" was driving the nation to ruin. And millions found their way to the Savior because of his witness and his preaching.

In the late 1800s, at age seven, he told his grandfather, "I'm going to hunt around and find a good job I can do with my head." He ended up as a center fielder for the Chicago, Pittsburgh, and Philadelphia professional baseball teams at a time when it was recognized as a sport populated largely by the socially challenged and others who could find no other viable means of financial support.

While on a weekend bender with a few of his teammates, he stumbled across the threshold of the Pacific Garden Mission in Chicago, and soon thereafter, the baseball world lost one of their most colorful players to a higher league and to a team whose legacy would be remembered far longer than any pennant drive. He enjoyed dramatizing his conversion: "Twenty-seven years ago I turned and left that little group on the corner of State and Van Buren Streets, walked into the little mission, fell on my knees, staggered out of sin, and into the arms of the Savior. If the same floor is in that old building, I can show you the knothole in the board upon which I knelt that dark and stormy night . . . I have followed Jesus from that day to this very second, like the hound on the trail of the fox, and will continue until he leads me through the pearly gate into the presence of God and it closes on its jeweled hinges."

It was not long before the irrepressible William "Billy" Ashley Sunday became the most talked about, the most revered, the most despised, and the most successful evangelist of all time. His preaching tours took him throughout America. Newspaper reporters would not leave him alone, and periodicals devoted seemingly endless columns to his sermons and preaching campaigns. As if they were using a hypodermic needle, the working press shot his message into the bloodstream of a nation that came by the thousands to hear him speak three and four times a day.

I have followed Jesus from that day to this very second, like the hound on the trail of the fox, and will continue until he leads me through the pearly gate into the presence of God and it closes on its jeweled hinges.

SURRENDER TO GOD'S SUPREMACY

Billy Sunday believed the Bible was the true Word of God and the force of life itself. He would preach to a spellbound audience, "And, oh, what a time we'll have in heaven. In heaven they never mar the hillsides with spades, for they dig no graves. In heaven they never telephone for the doctor, for nobody gets sick. In heaven no one carries handkerchiefs, for nobody cries." As he preached the uncompromising Word of God, he would declare that to know God meant for people to give their whole selves to God, to be crucified with Christ, to break their stubborn independence from

God, and to surrender to the supremacy of the One who loved them enough to die for them. Billy Sunday's influence was enormous during that era dubbed the Roaring Twenties when he would often capture center stage from many of the other luminaries of his day, such as Charles Lindbergh, Babe Ruth, Mae West, Charlie Chaplin, Mary Pickford, and Ernest Hemingway.

☀ The average church has so much machinery and so little oil of the Holy Spirit that it squeaks like a threshing machine when you start it up in the fall after it has been out in the field all the year.

He was such a gifted communicator that before long his memorable quotes were collected and called *Sundayisms*. Some of his most popular sayings included these:

- Sin flourishes because people treat it like a cream puff.

- I contend there should be some visible connection between the thing a man believes in and himself.

- A lot of churches don't need an evangelist as much as they need an undertaker.

- The average church has so much machinery and so little oil of the Holy Spirit that it squeaks like a threshing machine when you start it up in the fall after it has been out in the field all the year.

- Some preachers don't believe in revivals; neither does the devil.

- Some men are miserable because they have just enough religion to give them goose pimples.

- They tell me a revival is only temporary; so is a bath, but it does you good.

How did God use this man to help drive a raucous nation to its knees? Why did people swarm to the altar in tears and repentance for their sins? Why did they come in full surrender to Jesus Christ holding out no conditions, signing away all rights to their lives, breaking their independence from God, and choosing to become bondslaves to the Savior? God used Billy Sunday because he believed and lived out these words of the apostle: "I eagerly expect and hope that I will in no way be ashamed, but will have sufficient courage so that now as always Christ will be exalted in my body, whether by life or by death. For to me, to live is Christ and to die is gain" (Philippians 1:20–21).

Billy Sunday knew then what we all must know and implement now, if there is to be an outpouring of God's Spirit in our personal lives, in our churches, and in our nation: Only when there is a continual denial of self and full surrender to God will there be a growing willingness in our hearts to do what the Master is calling us to do. Until our minds and wills are called into order by the Spirit of God, they will remain open to every foreign idea, every theological aberration, and the acceptance of virtually anything that feels good, looks good, takes virtually no commitment, and has drive-in convenience. None of this will move us closer to God and into His presence.

Only when we lift our hands to the Father in full surrender to His will can we understand even remotely what God wants to do in our lives. And as we enter God's gateway to the supernatural, one of the most immediate messages we will receive from our holy God is, "My son, my daughter, are you prepared to surrender it all? To give up your shallow lives for an experience that will touch your heart for eternity? I will not tell you where I will have you go. I just want to know if you are prepared to surrender your life to Me. Each morning when you awake, I will be with you to help you and guide you through your day. But my question remains: As you do your daily duties, will you surrender it all . . . to Me."

WHAT IS REVIVAL?

Until we make a decision to deal honestly with God's questions about full allegiance to Him, there will be little or no prospect of an awakening in our hearts, no stirring of the Spirit in our churches, and no revival in our land. True revival is nothing less or more than the manifested presence of God in our lives. It is when Jesus is free to be who He wants to be in, through, and around us.

Billy Sunday preached this message as hard in his day as we need to communicate it in our day. With one foot off the ground and his arm piercing the air, he said this:

A revival does two things. First, it returns the Church from her backsliding and second, it causes the conversion of men and women; and it always includes the conviction of sin on the part of the Church. What a spell the devil seems to cast over the Church today. When is a revival needed? When the individuals are careless and unconcerned. If the Church were down on her face in prayer, they would be more concerned with the fellow outside. The Church has degenerated into a third-rate amusement joint, with religion left out. When is a revival needed? When carelessness and unconcern keep the people asleep. It is as much the duty of the Church to awaken and work and labor for the men and women of this city as it is the duty of the fire department to rush out when the call sounds. What would you think of the fire department if it slept while the town burned? You would condemn them. It is just as much your business to be awake. The Church of God is asleep today; it is turned into a dormitory, and has taken the devil's opiates.

Could not—should not—this message be preached throughout the land today? Or are we, perhaps, too sensitive, too sophisticated? Is Billy Sunday just an old-fashioned, fire-and-brimstone preacher who's out of date, out of touch, and whose message, we hope, stays out of sight? Are his words and his style too strong, too politically incorrect, too offensive for our less-tolerant sensibilities in these last days of the twentieth century? Are there other words and phrases we would rather use, perhaps, instead of *surrender, commitment, compelling vision?* Could it be we've not seen an all-out awakening because individual believers and our church leaders have failed to set themselves apart, and in humility and desperation surrender themselves fully to God?

The Scripture tells us that without a vision the people die. They die in spirit, in their influence, in right decision-making, in their zeal to share their faith with neighbors, and they die in their desire to bring closure to the Great Commission by keeping the gospel neat and tidy, homogenized and pasteurized, so there's no way a lost world could know of the unwrapped gift that awaits them. Until the Church of Jesus Christ regains its spiritual power, recaptures its spiritual passion, is willing to pay the price, and begins to demonstrate an unfailing love for Jesus Christ, it will remain cold, traditional, out of touch, ineffective, purposeless, nonproductive, ingrown, and something so tepid that the only sensible thing to do is to spit it out.

Harsh words, but this is where we are. Only an outpouring of God's Spirit that leads to revival will win the day.

A SACRIFICE OF YOUR FEELINGS

But Billy Sunday is not finished with us yet:

> When may a revival be expected? When the wickedness of the wicked grieves and distresses the Christian. Sometimes people don't seem to mind the sins of other people. Don't seem to mind while boys and girls walk the streets of their city and know more of evil than gray-haired men. You are asleep. When is a revival needed? When the Christians have lost the spirit of prayer.
>
> When may a revival be expected? When the wickedness of the wicked grieves and distresses the Church. When you are willing to make a sacrifice for the revival; when you are willing to sacrifice your feelings. You say, "Oh, well, Mr. Sunday hurt my feelings." Then don't spread them all over this tabernacle for men to walk on. Make a sacrifice of your feelings; make a sacrifice of your business, of your time, of your money; you are willing to give help to advance God's cause, for God's cause has to have money the same as a railroad or a steamship company. You give your influence and stand up and let people know you stand for Jesus Christ and it has your endorsement and time and money. Somebody has got to get on the firing line. Somebody has to be willing to make a sacrifice. They must be willing to get out and hustle and do things for God.

Second Chronicles 7:14 is God's ultimate blueprint for revival: "If my people, who are called by my name, will humble themselves and pray and seek my face and turn from their wicked ways, then will I hear from heaven and will forgive their sin and will heal their land." Revival will never come to the proud. It will only come to the hearts of those who've taken the initiative to humble their hearts before God, asking His forgiveness for past wrongs. Revival will never come to those who refuse to pray with repentant hearts. It will only come to those who are on their knees before God, confessing their sins, making amends for how they've treated others, and asking God to lead them in His ways and to think His thoughts. Revival will not come if we and our priorities are out of line. It will only come to those who seek *first* the kingdom of God; who seek *first* the face of Jesus; who seek *first* to know His counsel, and not rely on the spurious, fickle wisdom of man. Then, and only then, God says, will He bring healing to individuals, to our churches, and to our land. The good news is that *there is hope.* The answer is not just blowing randomly in the wind. The answer is real, bonafide, honest Truth. Our country is not in its present chaos because of left-wing liberals or the activities of right-wing radicals, but because of an insipid Christianity that refuses to take the Word of God seriously, and doesn't believe it's possible to have a deeper relationship with our heavenly Father. The church is lukewarm, and it needs to wake up *now* if there will ever be God's true anointing and a mighty, sweeping revival in our land.

When may a revival be expected? When the wickedness of the wicked grieves and distresses the Church. When you are willing to make a sacrifice for the revival; when you are willing to sacrifice your feelings.

TRANSFER OF OWNERSHIP

We will never choose to let God have His way with us if we continue to hang on to our own desires, our own dreams, and our own bondage. In wartime, if we are captured by an enemy, we are commanded to surrender. At that moment, we have a choice. We can take our chances, make a run for it, and hope for the best. But if an armed enemy pursues us, there is little chance of our physical survival. When God asks us to surrender to Him, the analogy is the same, except for one key point: God is not the enemy. He is our Father and our Friend. He knows what's best for us. That's why He wants us to surrender our minds to Him (the way we think); our wills (what we're convinced we should be or do); our emotions (how we feel); our bodies (the sum of who we are); our talents (the abilities for which *we* often take full credit); our attitudes (our often selfish responses to others); our motives (what we know *really* drives us to succeed); our careers (the business of life that too often *becomes* our life).

Surrender is all about a *transfer of ownership*—an exchanged life. And when we enter God's gateway to supernatural power for living we begin to learn what *an exchanged life* is all about. When we fast and pray we may become influenced by God's character. We may hear Him speak to us in a voice we've never heard before. It's not a harsh voice, but rather the voice of a waiting Father who will always tell us the truth. Whenever God calls me to fast, where I deny myself the natural act of eating to focus on specific spiritual goals, I ask God to show me those areas in my life that I'm still keeping for Ronnie Floyd, asking, "God, what am I still not surrendering fully to you? Show me. Instruct me. I cannot see the blind spots in my life without your divine counsel."

This time *I* will ask Billy Sunday's question: "When may a revival be expected?" It's when the alienation from God of those who surround us causes us so much distress that we are driven to our knees, asking for God's mercy, understanding, compassion, love, and forgiveness. The question is simply, "How often do we come before God with a repentant heart?" We sing the song, "I Surrender All," but under our breath intone, "but not really, God, at least *not right now.*" We pray, "Lord, Your will be done in my life," but we attach a hushed P.S. that says, "that is, unless it's too painful, demands too much, puts my life in jeopardy, or is too inconvenient." The singular condition of obtaining God's full blessing is complete, full, and absolute surrender. Thousands of hearts have said they'd do it. Thousands more have made the attempt. But most have failed miserably because they never discovered the supernatural power necessary to live such a life before God.

Andrew Murray writes in his sermon *Absolute Surrender,* that God is . . .

the Fountain of life, the only Source of existence and power and goodness, and throughout the universe there is nothing good but what God works. God has created the sun and the moon and the stars and the flowers and the trees and the grass; and are they not all absolutely surrendered to God? Do they not allow God to work in them just what He pleases? When God clothes the lily with its beauty, is it not yielded up, surrendered, given over to God as He works in its beauty? And God's redeemed children . . . can you think that God can work His work if there is only half or a part of them surrendered? God cannot do it. God is life and love and blessing and power and infinite beauty, and God delights to communicate Himself to every child who is prepared to receive Him. This one lack of absolute surrender is just the thing that hinders God. And now He comes, as God. He claims it.

TEMPORAL, BUT WITH LONG-LASTING EFFECT

Does a life of full surrender to God have its challenges? Yes, it does. The challenges and difficulties will be so overwhelming at times that we may want to retreat to our old ways of shaping our own destinies and running our own lives. That's why once we enter God's gateway to supernatural power we must never leave His presence. Fasting may be a temporal activity—a few days or forty days—but the significance and the effect of our fast and time with God is meant to last.

When asked if this full surrender is even possible, Andrew Murray responded, "What has God promised you, and what can God do to fill a vessel absolutely surrendered to Him? God wants to bless you in a way beyond what you expect. From the beginning, ear hath not heard, neither hath the eye seen what God hath prepared for them that wait for Him. God has prepared unheard of things you never can think of: blessings much more wonderful than you can imagine, more mighty than you can conceive. They are divine blessings."

If our lives are not receptive to the things of God, if it's business as usual, if our tempers rule us, our emotions control us, our minds deceive us, and our hearts are not warm to the God who loves us, I suggest that surrender to God has not yet become a viable activity in our lives. If that is the case, then our Christian walks will be most difficult assignments, bordering on confusion and drudgery, because we shall be wearing masks, playing charades, pretending to be one thing but, in truth, being quite the opposite. We fool only ourselves, and with each sleight of heart, we put more distance between ourselves and the God who loves us. We remain miserable when we depend on our own talents and make our own plans, becoming even more distressed when we then ask God to bless our homemade efforts, knowing He had no part in them.

When someone asked William Booth, founder of the Salvation Army, the secret of his enormous success, Booth remained silent for several moments. Finally, with tear-filled eyes, he said, "There have been men with greater brains or opportunities than I, but I made up my mind that God would have all of William Booth there was."

Several years later when General Booth's daughter heard about her father's comment regarding his full surrender to God, she said, "That wasn't really his secret—his secret was that he never took it back."

There is also a practical side to surrendering fully to God: Our burdens become His, not ours. Finally, we start to place our frustrations and worries where we once only laid our sins.

And that's the secret we need to discover: We may never be a William Booth, but all of us can, in response to God's grace and mercy in saving us, give Him our all—and never take it back. There is also a practical side to surrendering fully to God: Our burdens become His, not ours. Finally, we start to place our frustrations and worries where we once only laid our sins. We develop a spiritually healthy perspective on what was once a terrible frustration with life and its inconsistencies because we now no longer must carry the burden. Once filled with dark, foreboding thoughts, we now are free to be the people God created us to be because He has cast out those terrible demons of fear, anxiety, co-dependence, having to be number one, attitudes that hurt, and actions that are unkind. As we go into that quiet place to meet God in fasting and prayer, our souls are focused on Him alone, and therein lies the difference. We become oblivious to the noise of life when we are in His presence.

Life's babble is set aside as we throw ourselves at the feet of our Savior. It's only in the presence of our heavenly Father that we hear His call to full surrender.

FIVE DANGEROUS PRAYERS

Bill Hybels, a pastor and Christian leader, has suggested we consider five ideas for praying dangerously—prayers that will open us to God and cause us to want to stand in full surrender to Him. I encourage you to think these thoughts and pray these prayers as you put the cares of the world aside and enter God's presence in fasting and prayer. Here are Bill Hybels' five prayer challenges to us:

1. **Search me:** Almost every Christian has times of feeling indignant toward people who rebel against God. David expressed that emotion in Psalm 139, but immediately he stopped and asked God to examine him. In the same way, we must not forget to ask God to point out rebellion in our own spirits.

2. **Break me:** We cannot grow as Christians until we learn to ask for brokenness. Regardless of our level of spiritual maturity, there will always be areas of life in which God needs to work. Perhaps it's a penchant for perfectionism, an inclination to be discouraged, or stubborn insensitivity. Whatever it may be, new Christlike ways cannot replace the old until we let God smash the former patterns to bits.

3. **Stretch me:** This is the kind of prayer to pray when we want to grow up spiritually. When the first-century believers

prayed for greater boldness instead of asking God to take away persecution, they were praying stretch-me prayers. If we know people whose depth of love is humbling, whose perseverance is inspiring, whose spiritual strength is amazing, they have probably asked God to stretch them through life's challenges.

4. **Lead me:** Asking God to take our lives and do whatever He wants with them is risky. If we are comfortable in our homes, have growing families, and enjoy our jobs, it's especially scary to let God take control, but that's what faith is all about. We've got to believe that His plans for us are better than our own.

5. **Use me:** It's exciting to make ourselves available to God so that He can touch someone else through us. Such prayer creates adventures. [2]

To Bill Hybels' five prayers I would add *Teach me,* Lord to surrender. It is only through letting go that we will ever learn to live life as God meant it to be lived. Spiritual arrogance is one of the greatest detriments to God moving in the church today. Doctrine without spiritual power will only breed pride. One of the greatest attributes of a Spirit-controlled Christian is to be teachable to God and teachable to others. As a pastor, when I stand to share God's Truth with people, there inevitably will be some who will be so puffed up in spiritual arrogance that they are unwilling to learn. That's not the kind of spirit that prepares our hearts for revival. None of us ever arrives. A life of surrender to God must be characterized by praying for a teachable spirit. It's only through humility, when we admit we just don't know the answers, that we begin to grow as Christians.

Spiritual maturity is not a destination. Spiritual maturity is a journey. It's full surrender to God.

GOD IS ATTRACTED TO WEAKNESS

Surrender to God is to abandon all that we have to receive all that God possesses. It is not the skills, talents, and gifts that God places in our hands that matter, it is the full, complete, unequivocal surrender of those meager abilities to Him that He uses to do great things in our lives. In his wonderful book *Fresh Wind, Fresh Fire,* Jim Cymbala, pastor of the Brooklyn Tabernacle Church in Brooklyn, New York, wrote: "I discovered an astonishing truth; God is attracted to weakness. He can't resist those who humbly and honestly admit how desperately they need him. The first step in any spiritual awakening is demolition. We cannot make headway in seeking God without first tearing down the accumulated junk in our souls. Rationalizing has to cease. We have to start seeing the sinful debris we hadn't noticed before, which is what holds back the blessing of God. Sin grieves the Holy Spirit and quenches His power among us."

Surrender means we must be emptied before we can be filled. We must die to live; give it all up to gain. No great work anywhere by anyone at any time has ever come about without surrender. For His Kingdom to come, our kingdom must go.

In the words of Flora Larsson from *My Treasure Chest* . . .

> *Have it Your own way, Lord,*
> *You've won!*
> *I lay my weapons down.*
> *You would not give me blow for blow,*
> *No steel met mine,*
> *And yet I am vanquished.*

When we surrender to God, we become better promise keepers, better fathers, better mothers, better husbands, and better wives *because we have transferred our lives, our ideas, our best-laid plans over to our heavenly Father.* It's the transfer of our bodies (all we are); our minds (how we think); our spirits (where God lives); our tongues (every word we utter); our attitudes (the way we *respond* to others); and our motives (the reality of who we are). All that God has given us we must transfer, give over, *surrender* to Him for His great purposes, and no longer keep them for our own. The more we live in God's holy presence, staying focused on Him through the joys of the disciplines of fasting and prayer, the more we will learn of His character, and that's what we must desire more than life itself. No one has ever *made* more promises than God, no one has ever *kept* more promises than God, and no one has ever been more *faithful* than God. He knows that we are engaged in the battle of our lives, because He has already told us: "For our struggle is not against flesh and blood, but against the rulers, against the authorities, against the powers of this dark world and against the spiritual forces of evil in the heavenly realms. Therefore put on the full armor of God, so that when the day of evil comes, you may be able to stand your ground, and after you have done everything, to stand" (Ephesians 6:12–13).

MIGHTY MEN

In 1995 a member of my church, Dr. Jeff Rhodes, sent a special letter to thirty men in our congregation. The letter he wrote, and the ministry he started on my behalf, "Pastor's Mighty Men," comes from the heart of a man for whom fasting and prayer have become integral to his spiritual worship. Jeff was a committee of one to invite thirty godly men to "hold up their pastor's arms," and to be volunteers to support him in any way for spiritual warfare. This awareness came to him during one of his fasts when Jeff asked God specifically how he could be a special encouragement to his pastor. With Jeff's permission, I'm sharing with you his letter of invitation to those individuals invited to become the "Pastor's Mighty Men."

Dear Sir,

I am writing to you to ask if you would be interested in a new ministry that I am starting. The Lord has shown me the amount of demonic attack our pastor is undergoing. His very life is, at times, in peril. Therefore, I feel that the Lord has led me to develop a ministry of support and prayer for him. Pastor Floyd himself has discussed this with me and is very interested in having some type of additional support for our church, our pastor, our staff, and their families. He mentioned a church where the men fast and pray one day a year. However, I feel that we should organize ourselves differently. I am asking for thirty men to be warriors for the Lord on behalf of our Pastor and church. Each man will select a day of the month (first, fifteenth, etc.) and fast and pray on that date each month. We will use the standards set for deacons found in 1 Timothy and ask the Lord to direct us to specific men. It would be a grave error to ask a man who was not walking with God to stand in the gap for the church. If we have more than thirty men, we will begin to double up on days. I would like for us to begin in secret, and present ourselves to the Pastor on his birthday in mid-November. If you believe that you know someone who would make a good member of "Pastor's Mighty Men," please contact me, and I will send them a letter. The Lord has given me a vision that we get enough men to surround the sanctuary, holding hands, interceding on behalf of the Pastor and staff, asking the Holy Spirit to move in a mighty way—sort of a Temple Guard.

Please remember, this is warfare. You will be attacked for participating. Let's not shrink back, but rather push on toward the Lord's calling in our lives. Please be praying for each other as well. Always keep in mind, men who participate with wrong motives will not be able to stand. Only invite men to come and pray who are willing to stand in the gap.

In 1 Samuel 26:15–16 David said, "You're a man, aren't you? And who is like you in Israel? Why didn't you guard your [pastor]? Someone came to destroy your [pastor]. What you have done is not good. As surely as the LORD lives, you and your men deserve to die, because you did not guard your [leader], the LORD's anointed. . . ." Zechariah 10:7 reads, "The Ephraimites will become like mighty men, and their hearts will be glad as with wine. Their children will see it and be joyful; their hearts will rejoice in the LORD."

Dr. Jeff Rhodes

On my birthday, I received another letter from Jeff stating that "Pastor's Mighty Men" was now in place, with each man fasting and praying for me one day each month—meaning that one of God's choice men was fasting and praying for me every day of the year. Since its inception, "Pastor's Mighty Men" has not missed a day, and I have felt the supernatural power of my living God in ways I will never be able to describe. What the men are telling me is this: They have never felt the spiritual battle as strongly as they feel it today—both for me, and for themselves and their families. Their surrender to God to do what He would have them do has changed their lives, opened up creative avenues for witness, and has brought them, too, through God's gateway to supernatural power.

In *My Utmost for His Highest,* Oswald Chambers writes, "Is the mind of my spirit in perfect agreement with the life of the Son of God in me . . . ? I have the responsibility of keeping my spirit in agreement with His Spirit, and by degrees Jesus lifts me up to where He lived—in perfect consecration to His Father's will, paying no attention to any other thing . . . Is God getting His way with me, and are other people beginning to see God in my life more and more?" [3]

If those around us are seeing God through us because of our full surrender to Him and His cause, then something else will also begin to happen: We will become people who are more trustworthy, more responsible, and increasingly attentive to the spiritual, physical, and emotional needs of others. People will also begin to know we are Christians because of our love, our faith, and our being people who say what we mean and mean what we say—*keepers of our promises,* one of the greatest God-honoring hallmarks of His servants.

Why do you boast of evil . . . you who are a disgrace in the eyes of God? Your tongue plots destruction; it is like a sharpened razor . . . You love evil rather than good, falsehood rather than speaking the truth.

PSALM 52:1‒3

Your promises have been thoroughly tested, and your servant loves them.

PSALM 119:140

CHAPTER EIGHT

Keeping Our Promises to God

The glory of these forty days we celebrate with songs of praise;
for Christ, through whom all things were made,
himself has fasted and has prayed.

Alone and fasting Moses saw the loving God who gave the law;
And to Elijah, fasting, came the steeds and chariots of flame.
So Daniel trained his mystic sight, delivered from the lions' might;
and John, the Bridegroom's friend, became the herald of
   Messiah's name.

Then grant us, Lord,
like them to be full oft in fast and prayer with thee;
our spirits strength with thy grace, and give us joy to see thy face.
Father, Son, and Spirit blest, to thee be every prayer addressed,
who art in threefold Name adored, from age to age, the only Lord.[1]

THE GLORY OF THESE FORTY DAYS, or fourteen days, or one or two days, or one day each month—whenever we come into the presence of our living God in fasting and prayer—it will be a glorious experience. What may have been a perfunctory "I promise to love you, and serve you, Jesus" prayer in the past is now transformed from the dull routine of vain repetition to one of adoration, praise, confession, and thanksgiving as we present ourselves humbly before the King of Kings, asking

Him to direct our steps, control our thoughts, and warm our hearts. Once hastily spoken, and perhaps even bordering on the insincere, our more thoughtful promises to God now take on new significance: Our promises to be kinder, more loving, more in control of our tempers, more effective in our witness, better fathers, mothers, husbands, and wives echo in the purity of His presence.

SPECTATOR OR PLAYER?

Are the spiritual disciplines of fasting and praying necessary to see our promises to God in this new dimension? Are prayer and fasting mandatory? I'll answer this question with another question. If we wanted to become tennis players, would it be possible for us to participate in the game without hitting the ball and running to get the ball to return it? Some action must take place if we are to be *in the game.* Those who choose not to play the game are called spectators, lookers-on, involved to a degree, but only on the periphery, and away from the action. There's nothing wrong with being spectators—that is, *unless* they sit idly in the stands and watch only because they have not yet been informed that they, too, have been invited to play. God will not coax or wheedle us to accept the conditions necessary to enjoy the supernatural power He promises will be ours through fasting and prayer. But He has issued an invitation to what promises to be the experience of our lives. Fasting-and-prayer seasons are for reflection, celebration, and gratitude carried out in a spirit of quietness—an unseen, unnoticed activity, kept from the prying eyes of others, an experience to be enjoyed alone with God. This verse sets the tone for any fast we might undertake:

When you fast, do not look somber as the hypocrites do, for they disfigure their faces to show men they are fasting. I tell you the truth, they have received their reward in full. But when you fast, put oil on your head and wash your face, so that it will not be obvious to men that you are fasting, but only to your Father, who is unseen; and your Father, who sees what is done in secret, will reward you. (Matthew 6:16–18)

Fasting-and-prayer seasons are meant for reflection, celebration, and gratitude, carried out in a spirit of quietness—an unseen, unnoticed activity, kept from the prying eyes of others, an experience to be enjoyed alone with God.

SOUND THEOLOGY

When we fast and pray, our focus will always be on our heavenly Father. It must be God-directed, not us-directed. Nor is it a way to show the world that *we are righteous*. If that's our objective, we will be miserable indeed, and like the Pharisees, we will have already received our rewards in full. Instead, it's a way to bring clarity and focus to our spiritual eyes. It allows us to tunnel through the normal, insatiable desires of our bodies for food and other creature comforts to get to what a life in Christ is all about. We are so preoccupied with the sound and fury of *things* that we seldom move deep into the core of life itself, into that realm of our spirits that too easily lies hidden from the truth of God and the light of His love. Sadly, if we remain spectators—never entering the game— we may be obliged to live out our days without taking hold of God's best, never assimilating His nourishing power, and never putting our feet on the solid ground of God's great promises.

In a *Peanuts* cartoon strip, Lucy and Linus are staring out the window, watching it rain. The conversation goes like this:

Lucy: "Boy! Look at it pour. What if it floods the whole world?"

Linus: "It won't. In Genesis 9 God promised Noah that would never happen again. The sign of that promise is the rainbow."

Lucy, turning back to the window with a big smile: "You've taken a great load off my mind."

Linus: "Sound theology has a way of doing that."

Chuck Swindoll comments: "Wise and timely words from little Linus. With feelings of fear and uncertainty while watching events from our windows, many of us often hear least what we need most. Sound, reliable theology that offers reassurance and hope . . . based squarely on God's Word. Not feelings or opinions or even logic. We need to hear what God has said and rest our case there."[2]

When we make our promises to God in the light of His presence, we make them with new information, sound theology, and from a fundamentally new perspective. There are still many things we must do, but now we embrace a dramatic difference in how we see God's call on our lives. The promises we make no longer are made in our own self-interests, not to make us look good, nor to give us the appearances of being religious. Our promises are made to God. He is the One who will hold us accountable. Where we once esteemed ourselves as number one, winning is now no longer our primary objective; triumph at any cost and *on our terms* has been left at the foot of the cross; the former driving issues of self-actualization, personal fulfillment, self-love, and other subtle or overt demonstrations of narcissism are seen for what they are: shallow, shadowy disguises of what a life with God is meant to be.

THE AMERICAN DREAM REVISITED

As we experience God's supernatural power, our direction shifts to a concentration on things of the heart and to relationships that matter. But this change of direction will not come without paying a price. Fasting and prayer help quiet our spirits so we can tunnel through our cultural trappings, an insane political correctness, the tendency to go along with the crowd, and the godless values of our society, many of which have become so much a part of our personal lives and our churches that there is little or no difference from life outside. The highly touted, always elusive, but continually sought-after package called The American Dream is so tied to our ritualistic, cultural thinking that it has infiltrated our spiritual lives as well.

Momentarily, we may become concerned enough to organize a little prayer meeting and make some promises to God that we'll adjust the errors of our ways, after which we enjoy coffee and a donut. Then we change the subject abruptly and move to next week's ball game, the ups and downs of the Dow Jones average, what we think of our public officials, or whether we think the local bond issue will pass. There's nothing wrong with the group prayer meeting, the cup of coffee, the subject matter, or the fellowship. But they are not what will push us through God's gateway to supernatural power. We must do much more. No one can walk with God for us, and we never again need to live on or off the experiences of others. God will help us create our own experiences, and He will always create them in accordance to His Word. But for this to happen *we* must pursue God. When we simply tap lightly at the door of our hunger for God, not much of anything will ever happen in our spiritual lives. The encumbrances of life will remain so much baggage, but unbothered by its weight, we'll continue to carry it; the impenetrable walls of the distractions of daily living will never be scaled, and because of our familiarity with our prison, we no longer notice its lofty walls; the impediments of life itself will pull us down, keep us down, and prevent us from recognizing our desperate condition, making us unaware of our need to lift up our heads and cry out with the psalmist:

> Listen to my cry for help, my King and my God, for to you I pray. In the morning, O LORD, you hear my voice; in the morning I lay my requests before you and wait in expectation. (Psalm 5:2–3)

> Do not be far from me, for trouble is near and there is no one to help. (Psalm 22:11)

> But you, O LORD, be not far off; O my Strength, come quickly to help me. (Psalm 22:19)

> Hear my cry for mercy as I call to you for help, as I lift up my hands toward your Most Holy Place. (Psalm 28:2)

> Rise up and help us; redeem us because of your unfailing love. (Psalm 44:26)

A DETONATION OF AWARENESS

When we finally tire of going it alone, of living powerless lives, of taking little or no time to reflect on the condition of our relationships with God, of making promises we either cannot or do not intend to keep, when sitting in a pew is as close as we will get to God's presence, and when we sense our prayers make it about as far as the ceiling, then, perhaps, we will be desperate enough to call on God and ask Him to show us the way to His supernatural power.

When we see God as the only One who can remove the barriers of our unbelief, the only One who can give us the power we need for living, the only One who can create in us a new spirit, a new heart, and a new attitude, then we can move out of our spiritual darkness and enter the brilliant light of God's love.

New life from above bursts on our dead and darkened souls in what poet Calvin Miller calls a "detonation." In his book *A Hunger for Meaning*, Miller compares this to the experience of Helen Keller. He tells of the day when her teacher Anne Sullivan found the way to "unlock her silent blackness." Helen couldn't see or hear, so she had no way to learn sign language to communicate with signs or symbols. She had been touching hundreds of objects, but there seemed to be no way for her to know what they were. The discovery of communication came to Helen when her teacher took her to the well-house. Anne let cold water run over one of Helen's hands. In the other hand Anne formed the letters W-A-T-E-R in sign language.

Miller explains what happened next. "Suddenly Helen felt a symbol of something stirring in the gray darkness of her consciousness. Suddenly she came alive. She had a single word composed of five letters. But that single word of five letters set her free at last from the dumb prison of herself. Suddenly she knew that everything in the world had a name. She left the well-house alive with the new possibility of becoming a real, communicating person in a world that opened to her all at once."

We finally begin to understand that He wants us to reflect His glory and radiance in all areas of our lives, just as the moon, without a light source of its own, must rely on the sun for its brightness.

This is what can also happen to us when we enter the presence of God: We become alive with new possibilities, recognizing there really is more to life than news, standard-fare religion, weather, and sports. We will no longer ring a bell and expect God to appear as a heavenly bellhop, asking us how He can serve us. Living *in* Him and *through* Him means we will no longer treat Him as a casual visitor in our lives, appearing suddenly for an hour on Sunday only to vanish for the rest of the week. He now becomes a twenty-four-hour-a-day God. We are His, and He is ours. We finally begin to understand that He wants us to reflect His glory and radiance in all areas of our lives, just as the moon, without a light source of its own, must rely on the sun for its brightness.

REFLECTING GOD'S GLORY

One of the most practical theologians on the scene today is R. C. Sproul, chairman of the board for Ligonier Ministries. He has written such a poignant piece on the glory of God that I quote him at length. Dr. Sproul writes,

> When Moses went up on Mount Sinai to receive the Ten Commandments, the mountain was covered by God's presence in the form of His glory cloud. When he ascended the mountain Moses was swallowed up into this cloud. The people waited below for forty days, growing increasingly apprehensive because God had been angry with them over the golden calf incident, and fearful lest God destroy Moses.
>
> Meanwhile, Moses was talking with God on the mountain. Before he went up, Moses had made a bold request

of God, "Now show me your glory" (Exodus 33:18). God had replied something like, "Moses, you know that's impossible. No man can see me and live. But I will put you in the cleft of a rock and cover you with my hand. When I remove my hand you will see my back; but my face must not be seen."

So Moses got a *glance* at the *refracted* glory of the *back* of God. And what happened? When he came down from the mountain and the people saw him approaching in the distance they rushed forward to greet him. Then suddenly they shrank back in fear and cried out, "Moses, cover your face!" They were afraid to look at him, because the glory streaming from his face was blinding—glory shining from the face of a sinner who had seen the merest shadow of God's glory for one instant.

What was this glory? Notice that when God passed by Moses he pronounced these words: "The LORD, the LORD, the compassionate and gracious God, slow to anger, abounding in love and faithfulness, maintaining love to thousands, and forgiving wickedness, rebellion and sin. Yet he does not leave the guilty unpunished; he punishes the children and their children for the sin of the fathers to the third and fourth generation" (34:6-7). God's glory is not just overpowering; it is also holy."[3]

Exodus 34:29 says, "When Moses came down from Mount Sinai with the two tablets of the Testimony in his hands, he was not aware that his face was radiant because he had spoken with the LORD." This is what happens to us when we fast and pray with repentant, humble, contrite hearts. We focus on our time with God, but His radiance touches us forever, often without our knowing it. We simply realize that something supernatural has happened. We've been changed. Our priorities are no longer the same, and we know it will never be the same with God again. We now have divine protection and strength to do His will and to keep our promises to Him and to those around us. It's important to remember that it was through the experience of fasting and prayer that God gave Moses the Ten Commandments—our ten guidelines for life—commands and demands that He makes on His people. Could it be that we are only *in the lane* of being able to keep those promises when we are faithfully in the presence of God through fasting and prayer?

FASHIONED INTO PEOPLE OF INTEGRITY

Jesus, by His example and teaching, demonstrates that prayer and fasting are integral ingredients in the lives of His followers, with one of its primary purposes to bring our hearts to a place where we are fashioned into people of integrity, where we make promises, keep them, and become trustworthy people whose word is our bond. True fasting always draws us closer to God and His purposes. People often ask me why I think God chose prayer and fasting as the avenue to His supernatural power. I don't know the answer. I do know, however, that Scripture, prayer, and fasting are God's ways for believers to humble themselves in the sight of the Lord. I know of no other way to get close to the heart of God. When we humble ourselves in the sight of the Lord, He promises to exalt and lift us up at the appointed time (1 Peter 5:8–10; James 4:10). God also promises that He will resist the proud, but will give grace to the humble (James 4:6).

> ✴ **When we humble ourselves in the sight of the Lord, He promises to exalt and lift us up at the appointed time.**

Fasting brings sharp focus to the differences between our physical and spiritual natures. Eating is one of the most basic things we do as physical beings. One of our bodies' most natural desires is food. Without proper nourishment we die. By depriving ourselves of food for a spiritual purpose, we acknowledge our spiritual natures and honor our Creator-Father. When we deny the natural for the purpose of calling on God to do the supernatural, He enables and empowers us to experience His supernatural power. Through fasting, we confirm the words spoken by Jesus in the face of temptation during His forty-day fast: "Man does not live on bread alone, but on every word that comes from the mouth of God" (Matthew 4:4). Through prayer and fasting we forsake our own physical devices and the conveniences of this world and, instead, acknowledge and call upon God as Originator, Giver, Source, and Sustainer of all life, especially our own. He is raised up and praised as our hope and salvation. True spiritual fasting will result in submission, yielding ourselves to Him in love and devotion, making us people who speak the truth because we have been with God.

God's Word promises us His blessing when our fast . . .

- focuses on God and honors Him alone.

- has certain specific spiritual purposes to take us to the next level of our relationships with the Father.

- causes us to humble ourselves and submit to the authority of God and His Word.

- compels us to acknowledge and repent of sin in our lives.

- removes our natural bents toward self-worship to focus on spiritual goals and objectives.

- reminds us of the promises we have made to God and to those around us and that keeping those promises is a sign of our commitment to personal integrity.

> ✺ **It takes time to build character and a life of integrity, and we will not build it well without spending time in the holy presence of God.**

PASSING THE BATON OF TRUTH

Fasting and praying also give us strength for the long-haul. Life is not a sprint, it's a marathon. It takes time to build character and a life of integrity, and we will not build it well without spending time in the holy presence of God. Edith Schaeffer, in her book *What Is a Family?*, speaks of the relationship between family members as a "perpetual relay of truth." But her words, slightly modified here, extend far beyond the physical family and into every area of our lives—lives that are a series of relay races with a thousand batons to be passed on:

- *Determination*—sticking with the goods regardless

- *Honesty*—speaking and living the truth always

- *Responsibility*—being dependable and trustworthy

- *Thoughtfulness*—thinking of others before thinking of ourselves

- *Self-control*—staying calm under stress.

- *Patience*—fighting irritability; being willing to wait
- *Purity*—rejecting anything that lowers our standards
- *Compassion*—when others hurt, feeling their pain
- *Diligence*—working hard; toughing it out

But none of this can occur in our own strength. We become effective in our lives, with the right kind of godly influence, only when we walk under, into, and finally through God's gateway to supernatural power, knowing that, "He is the Rock, his works are perfect, and all his ways are just. A faithful God who does no wrong, upright and just is he" (Deuteronomy 32:4).

Dr. James Dobson also has something to say about batons as they relate to passing on God's values to His family. He writes, "According to the Christian values which govern my own life, my most important reason for living is to get the baton—the gospel—safely in the hands of my children. Of course, I want to place it in as many other hands as possible, and I'm deeply devoted to the ministry to families that God has given me. *Nevertheless, my number one responsibility is to evangelize my own children.* There is no higher calling on the face of the earth."[4]

PERSONAL WORD ON PASSING THE BATON

Before we can pass the baton of truth and promise-keeping to our families, colleagues, and others, we must remain in the presence of God long enough to have it given to us. If we don't receive the baton, we will have nothing to hand off. The good news is that our God promises to be with us throughout this marathon called life, whether we drop the baton or pass it on successfully to another. To run the race well we must enjoy the active presence of our heavenly Father during good times and bad.

AWAKEN AMERICA!

In 1995, God once again led me to fast and pray, and one of the tangible qualities that came from that fast was that God led me to give leadership to something we call Awaken America. Awaken America is a ministry that several of us take across the country—a team composed of my colleague, friend, and Worship Leader, Buster Pray, seven to twelve singers and band members, and me. We travel throughout the nation doing one-night meetings simply called Awaken America rallies. The purpose of our meetings is to call the church of Jesus Christ to repentance and to spiritual renewal.

Over these past months, we've observed that the more multidenominational, multicultural, multiracial and multiethnic these rallies are, the more the power of God is demonstrated among us. The message is becoming loud and clear: God is calling His Body into oneness. To God there is no such thing as Methodists, Catholics, Baptists, Pentecostals, Presbyterians, Assemblies of God, or nondenominational churches. When we come to Christ, we are part of His Body, without the attendant artificial divisions. That's why Ephesians 4:4 says that we need to have *one body,* if we are going to have any effect in our world.

WILL YOU TAKE THE BATON?

It seemed that in that first forty-day fast, God handed me a baton and said, "Ronnie Floyd, you have come to Me, and now I'm coming to you, asking you to call the American Church to awakening and spiritual renewal." I know this message that came to my heart from the heart of God is so that people everywhere—of every race, culture, denomination, and theological persuasion—will know they are *all* needed if we are to see closure to the Great

Commission and be awakened to the millions of unreached people in this generation.

One of the most profound moments in our meetings is our ministry time for their pastors, staff members, and their spouses. In that brief, ten-minute time together, we remind them that when the service is over, our small group will once again board an airplane and return to our homes. But before we leave, we share with them that it's our spiritual privilege and obligation to pass the baton on to them, and how important it is for them to realize it's now their duties to pray for a spiritual awakening in their own lives and in their churches. We remind them that if pastors, church staff members, and the lay leadership of our churches don't choose to take the baton, and humbly present themselves before God in prayer and fasting, we will never see a spiritual awakening in America. At the conclusion of that brief charge, we ask them to get on their knees and let our team and members of their own congregations come and pray for them.

Once God moves us into this part of the meeting, the awareness of everyone's need for a personal spiritual awakening seems to move to a new level. As God continues to lead me to conduct these meetings around the country, I promise to be faithful to God with the baton He has placed in my hand. But it's no good if it never *leaves* my hand—any more than with a runner in a relay race who never releases the baton to the next runner. It just wouldn't make sense! It's that release that makes it the kind of race it is. God has handed me this baton of prayer and fasting to hand on to you through this book. Writing this book has been an exercise in baton-passing. I'm handing it off to you. Will you receive it? Will you take it? Will you run with it? Will you fast and pray and be everything God wants you to be? If you take it, you'll need to become a person filled with credibility and integrity as never before, your life marked by keeping the promises we make to God, our families, our business associates, and all the relationships in our lives.

> ✳ **If we fail to trust Him, refuse to listen to His counsel, and thwart His direction for our lives, we will bring misery and despair upon ourselves, and there will be no help for us.**

When we praise and glorify Him, despite negative circumstances, we affirm His power and victory over our challenges. All things are possible with our God, but not all things will be easy. We may not understand how God is working in us at the outset, but once we catch a glimpse of His power, we see through a darkened glass no longer. His glory illuminates our hearts, and at that moment we forget about our lives as duty, instead responding to God and those around us from a heartfelt love, openness, and compassion because we have been standing on holy ground. We will keep our promises. We will make the commitment to deal only in truth. And even when we have done our best to keep our word, and we have accomplished all the Master has asked us to do, we will still be unprofitable servants in the light of His righteousness. If we fail to trust Him, refuse to listen to His counsel, and thwart His direction for our lives, we will bring misery and despair upon ourselves, and there will be no help for us. But as we allow Him to take control, and when we release the power of our own wills and emotions, our lives will be transfigured into hope, peace, and joy.

A. W. Tozer wrote, "True Christian joy is the heart's harmonious response to the Lord's song of love." That song of love includes the poetry of fasting and prayer, God-ordained vehicles to put us in the presence of our heavenly Father in a way we otherwise may never have known Him. That same Father is waiting to shower His power on those who love Him, who have made the bold promise to do their Savior's will, and whose faith is so strong they believe they can move mountains.

THE BOTTOM LINE

When we fast and pray, we practice the presence of God. He is holy. His character is impeccable. Just as His character rubbed off on a man named Moses, that same character—character that has as its hallmark *promise keeping*—will rub off on us as we come into His presence. Therefore, it's impossible to fast and pray and *not* keep the promises we make to God and others. In fact, if we don't keep our promises, it's a strong indication that we're not practicing the presence of God. We're not taking the time to be still and know that He alone is God.

One of the missing ingredients in the American church, and in the lives of thousands of Christians throughout our nation, is the lack of a genuine, holy fear of God. Promise breakers don't fear God. Promise keepers are those who fear God with such intensity and passion that when they fast and pray, God leads them to make new decisions and new promises *that they intend to keep*. There's a shortage of character in our land only because there's a shortage of the fear of God in our hearts.

In *Three Sisters,* Act III, the Russian playwright Anton Chekhov has Masha say,

> "I think a human being has got to have some faith, or at least he's got to seek faith. Otherwise his life will be empty, empty . . . How can you live and not know why the cranes fly, why children are born, why the stars shine in the sky!

. . . You must either know why you live, or else . . . nothing matters . . . everything's just wild grass."

. . . or hay, or stubble, or something of so little value that it's destined to be stomped on, not taken seriously, and ultimately destroyed. That's why we need the faith and encouragement to allow the spiritual experience of prayer and fasting to permeate every area of our daily lives, taking it out of the realm of the theoretical, and bringing it down to earth where we live, move, and have our being. Will you ask God if He is calling you to a fast in order to pray through any number of specific spiritual goals you may have for your life?

Before you read any further, this would be a good time to begin a prayer journal that will become a map of your spiritual journey. It will symbolize your commitment to want God's best for your life, along with a fresh, new, alive relationship with your heavenly Father that can begin when you enter His gateway to supernatural power. The outcome of your experience may lead you to learn to fast from judging others, to fast from anger and words that pollute, or perhaps to learn to fast from problems so great that they may be overwhelming you, driving you to despair.

O LORD, do not rebuke me in your anger or discipline me in your wrath. For your arrows have pierced me, and your hand has come down upon me.

PSALM 38:1–2

Blessed is the man you discipline, O LORD, the man you teach from your law; for the Lord will not reject his people; he will never forsake his inheritance.

PSALM 94:12, 14

CHAPTER NINE
Practicing the Disciplines of God

HE BEGAN HIS LIFE with all the classic handicaps and disadvantages. His mother was a powerfully built, dominating woman who found it difficult to love anyone. She had been married three times, and her second husband divorced her because she beat him up regularly. The father of the child I'm describing was her third husband; he died of a heart attack a few months before the child's birth. As a consequence, the mother had to work long hours from his earliest childhood.

She gave him no affection, no love, no discipline, and no training during those early years. She even forbade him to call her at work. Other children had little to do with him; so he was alone most of the time. He was ugly and poor and untrained and unlovable. When he was thirteen years old, a school psychologist commented that he probably didn't even know the meaning of the word love. During adolescence, the girls would have nothing to do with him and he fought with the boys.

He thought he might find a new acceptance in the Marine Corps; they reportedly built men, and he wanted to be one. But his problems went with him.

Despite a high IQ, he failed academically and finally dropped out during his third year of high school. He thought he might find a new acceptance in the Marine Corps; they reportedly built men, and he wanted to be one. But his problems went with him. The other Marines laughed at him and ridiculed him. He fought back, resisted authority, and was court-martialed and thrown out of the Marines with an dishonorable discharge. So there he was—a young man in his early twenties—absolutely friendless and shipwrecked. He was small and scrawny in stature. He had an adolescent squeak in his voice. He was balding. He had no talent, no skill, no sense of worthiness. He didn't even have a driver's license.

Once again he thought he could run from his problems, so he went to live in a foreign country. But he was rejected there too. Nothing had changed. While there, he married a girl who herself had been an illegitimate child and brought her back to America with him. Soon, she began to develop the same contempt for him that everyone else displayed. She bore him two children, but he never enjoyed the status and respect that a father should have. His marriage continued to crumble. His wife demanded more and more things that he could not provide. Instead of being his ally against the bitter world, as he had hoped, she became his most vicious opponent. She could outfight him, and she learned to bully him. On one occasion, she locked him in the bathroom as punishment. Finally, she forced him to leave.

PRIVATE NIGHTMARE

He tried to make it on his own, but he was terribly lonely. After days of solitude, he went home and literally begged her to take him back. He surrendered all pride. He crawled. He accepted humiliation. He came on her terms. Despite his meager salary, he brought her seventy-eight dollars as a gift, asking her to take it and spend it any way she wished. But she laughed at him. She belittled his feeble attempts to supply the family's needs. She ridiculed his failure and made fun of his sexual impotency in front of a friend who was there. At one point, he fell on his knees and wept bitterly, as the greater darkness of his private nightmare enveloped him.

No one wanted him. No one had ever wanted him. He was perhaps the most rejected man of our time. His ego lay shattered in fragmented dust!

Finally, in silence, he pleaded no more. No one wanted him. No one had ever wanted him. He was perhaps the most rejected man of our time. His ego lay shattered in fragmented dust! The next day, he was a strangely different man. He arose, went to the garage, and took down a rifle he had hidden there. He carried it with him to his newly acquired job at a book-storage building. And from a window on the third floor of that building, shortly after noon, November 22, 1963, he sent two shells crashing into the head of President John Fitzgerald Kennedy.[1]

Whenever I read this chilling account of how Lee Harvey Oswald grew up friendless, judged, angry, and his mind polluted with hate and suspicion, a chill runs up and down my spine. A twenty-four-year-old Oswald was an explosion waiting to happen, and happen it did on that late Dallas morning. A unique story? Yes, in that he assassinated a president of the United States. But beyond that, it's all too common. His tortured life reminds me that we also treat people—often those closest to us—in ways they do not deserve to be treated. When we abuse people physically or emotionally, we create such trauma in their lives that they may actually somaticize their sickness, turning it from an emotional malady into an actual physical illness. When we allow our negativity to crush someone's long-desired dream and permit our gossip and anger to ruin reputations, we *will* pay in the end . . . somehow. Our sharp, cutting tongues are not necessarily indicators of keen minds, and repentance is not only saying "I'm sorry," but it's also saying "I'm through." Only God and we know if we stand guilty of these charges.

ONE TOO MANY

Even one act of emotional abuse is too much. To damage the gentle spirit of just one child is a crime. To pollute only one person's mind with pornography, centerfolds, Internet sex, and other material that appeals to prurient interests is to infect the life of one too many. There may well be another Lee Harvey Oswald in some run-down apartment in your city or mine, opening up boxes of ammo and polishing a rifle, determining to get noticed one way or another, working up a final chance to say "Here I am, look at me!"

True fasting cannot, must not, be an inconsequential, intangible, theoretical, theological pursuit. Entering God's gateway to supernatural power needs to be more than a quiet spiritual journey to the heart of God.

These are tough words to begin a chapter in a book on fasting and prayer, but they are important words. As we look at the disciplines that God demands for the lives of His people, they line up with what you have just read. True fasting cannot, must not, be an inconsequential, intangible, theoretical, theological pursuit. Entering God's gateway to supernatural power needs to be more than a quiet spiritual journey to the heart of God. Our encounters with the Father must have an impact on every area of our lives—where we work, worship, play, and where we spend time with the people we love.

THE FIVE DISCIPLINES

Five specific *disciplines* can sure make major differences in our lives. As we work through these thoughts, we must look deeply into our hearts, asking God to remove any wickedness that might separate us from His presence. It would be inappropriate for me to suggest which areas are challenges to you, if any. It's only my prayer that God will use these thoughts to awaken our tired spirits and bring them closer to Him. We will explore each discipline as *a problem, a promise, and a prayer.*

Discipline 1: Fast from judging others; feast on Christ dwelling in them.

A Problem

The Inquisition, the Salem witch trials of Massachusetts, anti-Semitism, the oppression of minorities, the evils of racism, criticism of how people dress . . . these are all shallow indications that we are people who feel we have a right to judge others for who they are and what they do. We have become thoroughly skilled in passing judgment on people and issues that are inherently neither good nor bad, right nor wrong, even though we have been cautioned against serving as judge, jury, and executioner.

In the apostle Paul's day, one such divisive issue in the church was what to eat and not eat (Colossians 2:16). Today's challenges will differ greatly, but God's principle remains the same: When God's Word is silent, it is also *our* obligation to be silent. When we speak with a harsh and critical spirit, we are no better than the ungrateful steward in Matthew 18 who refused to wipe out an insignificant debt, even after he'd been forgiven a much larger one. If we would be forgiven, we must not judge, and we must also forgive.

A Promise

- For at whatever point you judge the other, you are condemning yourself, because you who pass judgment do the same things. (Romans 2:1)

- You, then, why do you judge your brother? Or why do you look down on your brother? For we will all stand before God's judgment seat. (Romans 14:10)

- Do not judge, and you will not be judged. Do not condemn, and you will not be condemned. Forgive, and you will be forgiven. (Luke 6:37)

A Prayer

God, in Your mercy, bring us close to Your heart. Help us realize that You are the final judge in all matters, and that setting ourselves up as lords over others is not our assignment. As we enter Your divine presence in fasting and prayer, we ask You to give us a clarity of mind and spirit that permits us to hear You when You speak to us at our greatest point of need: Forgive us for judging those we love. Forgive our insensitive hearts. In humility and sorrow, we commit ourselves to fast from judging others, and to feast on Christ dwelling in them. For Jesus' sake, Amen.

Discipline 2: Fast from fear of illness; feast on the healing power of God.

A Problem

We are human. We are prone to sickness and disease. For some of us, even the possibility of sickness makes us so fearful that we become immobilized, unable to work, even unable to pray. But it's in our fears where we meet ourselves. And what do we see? Often, we make the assumption that we must make ourselves healthy, that only medical assistance will see us through our crisis, that God really can't do much about our condition, and that, unfortunately, we're left to fend for ourselves. Where do we get these false thoughts? Not from Scripture. Not from our heavenly Father. In our sickness, God continually invites us to rely and concentrate on His supernatural power to heal our bodies, refresh our souls, and bring lasting peace to our troubled minds. That's the nature of our Father.

A Promise

- Then your light will break forth like the dawn, and your healing will quickly appear. (Isaiah 58:8)

- Pleasant words are a honeycomb, sweet to the soul and healing to the bones. (Proverbs 16:24)

- See now that I myself am He! There is no god besides me. I put to death and I bring to life, I have wounded and I will heal, and no one can deliver out of my hand. (Deuteronomy 32:39)

- If my people, who are called by my name, will humble themselves and pray and seek my face and turn from their wicked ways, then will I hear from heaven and will forgive their sin and will heal their land. (2 Chronicles 7:14)

A Prayer

In our weakness we enter Your presence, heavenly Father, asking You to help us focus on giving our whole selves to You—our minds, our emotions, and our bodies, when they are healthy and when they are sick. As we fast and pray for our healing and the healing of others, search our hearts, know our thoughts, cleanse us, and make us new. Help us to ask You the right questions—the ones that matter—and then may we wait patiently for Your answers. We humbly ask You to help us fast from all fear of illness, and to learn to feast on your mighty, supernatural, healing power. In Your holy name, Amen.

Discipline 3: Fast from words that pollute; feast on speech that purifies.

A Problem

Dirty air pollutes our lungs; unkind words pollute our hearts. Some say it goes even deeper, that we actually have developed an increasing loss of respect for public spaces and for the people who occupy those spaces. It happens in our homes, on the job, and on our highways. One poll found that 38 percent of Southern Californians admitted having made an obscene gesture at another driver, and one out of five had run a red light in the past month.

Why are we so rude to each other? Is it the breakneck pace of modern life? Too much violence in the media? Too great an eagerness to snatch a piece of the American Dream, even if it must come at a terrible price? I'm confident that much of the reason for our verbal abuse can be directed to the cataclysmic changes that have occurred in the American home. Married couples with children made up 44 percent of all households in the United

States in the sixties. Today, that figure has shrunk to less than 25 percent. The resulting increase of single-parent families is exacerbated by the rise of two-income households. Both trends mean there's almost no one around to tell and demonstrate to our children how to be courteous and how to use language that is uplifting and kind. Someone has said, "When moms went to work, the moral compass at home lost its magnetic north."

Unless an awakening to God occurs in our individual hearts, unless a revival of wholesome speech breaks out in our churches and communities, and unless an outpouring of God's Spirit helps us put *civil* back in *civilization,* our speech can and will only become further polluted, creating a nightmare of rudeness for generations to come.

A Promise
- The words of the wicked lie in wait for blood, but the speech of the upright rescues them. (Proverbs 12:6)

- He who loves a pure heart and whose speech is gracious will have the king for his friend. (Proverbs 22:11)

- Rather, as servants of God we commend ourselves in every way: in great endurance; in troubles, hardships and distresses; in truthful speech and in the power of God. (2 Corinthians 6:4, 7)

A Prayer
Almighty Father, teach us to speak Your Words. May our hearts be so infused with Your divine vocabulary that we will see our rudeness to others for the sin it is. As we set aside periods of time to fast and pray, may it be one of our objectives to have You teach us to speak

kindly to one another, to be patient with our spouses and our children, not to demand that we be number one at the office, and that we put others before us in word and in deed. We know You hear our prayers, Father. In the days ahead, please help us to remember we prayed it. Work in us the grace of obedience that will empower us to make our speech worthy of the lips You gave us. Help us fast from words that pollute, and give us the strength to feast on speech that purifies. In praise to You, O God, Amen.

Discipline 4: Fast from discontent; feast on gratitude.

A Problem

Half of the most unhappy people in the world are those individuals who didn't get what they wanted. The other half got what they thought they could not live without, only to discover it was not what they had in mind. The secret to a life of satisfaction and joy is not to sweat and strain for what we so passionately desire, but to live humbly with grateful hearts before our heavenly Father, fully at peace with what we already have. If we choose to live other than God's way, one day we'll discover the curtain on our earthly life has finally descended, and that we have missed the beauty and essence of life itself.

A Promise

- But godliness with contentment is great gain. For we brought nothing into the world, and we can take nothing out of it. (1 Timothy 6:6–7)

- For the love of money is a root of all kinds of evil. Some people, eager for money, have wandered from the faith and pierced themselves with many griefs. But you, man of God, flee from all this, and pursue righteousness, godliness, faith, love, endurance and gentleness. (1 Timothy 6:10–11)

- If they obey and serve him, they will spend the rest of their days in prosperity and their years in contentment. (Job 36:11)

A Prayer

Loving God, it is so obvious that we have no power whatever to help ourselves. Our sinful nature bends us toward discontentment, wanting more than we have, and envying those who possess what we feel we need. Forgive our selfish hearts, O Father. As we come to You respectfully and with repentant spirits in fasting and prayer, may You give us such a sharp focus that we will think Your thoughts, be content with Your miraculous ways, and trust You to help us abandon our consumer mentality and place our confidence in You alone. Keep us still before You, and help us to respond with our deeds and actions to all You have to tell us today. Lord, give us the courage to fast from our discontentment and help us to feast on gratitude for all You continue to do in our lives. In adoration and praise to You, Amen.

Discipline 5: Fast from problems that overwhelm; feast on prayer that sustains.

A Problem

About one in four Americans (26 percent) thinks the world will be in better shape in the year 2000 than it is now. Slightly more (27 percent) think it will be about the same, but 42 percent think the planet will be worse off by the turn of the century. Problems. They are like noses and ears—we all have them. Cold comfort rings out from the wings, "Hang in there." "Don't give up the ship." "Don't quit now." Inside we've already determined that our problems are too heavy for us to bear; overwhelmed, we enter periods of depression, with no sign of a solution to life's dilemmas. Our compulsion to control our own destinies finally gives in to an awareness that we may not make it after all. But the good news is that we are not in control, were never in control in the past, and will never be in control in the future. That's God's business. We are simply called to be faithful servants, and not to beat ourselves up over our imperfections.

Booker T. Washington said, "No man should be pitied because every day of his life he faces a hard, stubborn problem. It is the man who has no problems to solve, no hardships to face, who is to be pitied. He has nothing in his life which will strengthen and form his character, nothing to call out his latent powers and deepen and widen his hold on life."

So we have problems? Challenges? Opportunities? Our response to them depends on whether or not we view life from God's perspective—something we will never be able to accomplish if we refuse to slow down for periods of solitude, meditation, fasting, and prayer in the presence of our heavenly Father.

A Promise

- I have told you these things, so that in me you may have peace. In this world you will have trouble. But take heart! I have overcome the world." (John 16:33)

- Carry each other's burdens, and in this way you will fulfill the law of Christ. (Galatians 6:2)

- "They will fight against you but will not overcome you, for I am with you and will rescue you," declares the LORD. (Jeremiah 1:19)

A Prayer

> Father, it's sometimes so hard to see Your face because we have placed mounds of problems in front of You. But today, with Your strength, we will look for You in each obstacle, in every challenge. We need Your help, and we anticipate Your coming to us, because we need You every minute, every hour. As we fast and pray, help us to be dominated by Your presence, not by our problems; by Your love, not by our worries; by Your great promises, not by our anxieties. In Your strength, and by Your mighty hand, give us the wisdom to fast from problems that overwhelm us, and grant us Your grace to feast on prayer that sustains our hungry hearts. Amen.

As we walk through this life-changing gateway to supernatural power through God's call to prayer and fasting, I hope we will add to this list of areas where God may want to work in our lives. We may choose to begin with the following as God gives us strength to . . .

- fast from anger; feast on patience.
- fast from self-concern; feast on compassion.
- fast from suspicion; feast on truth.
- fast from gossip; feast on purposeful silence.
- fast from worry; feast on faith.

We have been created for something vastly more complex and profound than three daily meals, drink, clothing, and our hard-fought-for creature comforts.

NOT MY WILL

We can only wonder what the future of Lee Harvey Oswald might have been if those who raised him had fasted from anger and feasted on patience, and had fasted from suspicion and feasted on truth. I'm confident his story would have had a different, happier ending. Oswald's story is history, but you and I continue to exercise the option of choosing this day what, where, and whom we will serve. Will it be a fast from the lusts and colorful attractions that accompany the worst of our self-worship, giving tacit allegiance to the enemy who promises everything and delivers nothing? Or will we feast on serving a living God, entering His glorious presence, expecting His power to overwhelm us, His mercy to change us, and His love to make us whole? The choice is ours . . . today.

When we fast and pray, we are also bringing to the Lord the Lee Harvey Oswalds of this world—people who have never had a genuine relationship with or passion for the person of Jesus Christ. Fasting and praying is our time to listen to God. To assert our own wills in opposition to the holy mind of Christ is not merely wrong, it is high treason. That's why fasting and praying must also sensitize our spirits for those who are lonely, lost, dying, and without a Savior to bring sanity to their lives. Fasting and prayer can never be—must never be—an exercise for ourselves alone, nor does God want ecstatic dreamers who live only in the realm of the theoretical. Fasting and prayer must connect us with the bigger picture of God's full and complete redemption for mankind, which means He is giving us the privilege of being part of the magnificent finale to the Great Commission.

We have been created for something vastly more complex and profound than three daily meals, drink, clothing, and our hard-fought-for creature comforts. Yet that's where so much of our present and future continue to lie. But this is not all there is. God is waiting to give us His best, and He waits patiently for us to move through His gateway to supernatural power.

What anxiety are you prepared to release to Your heavenly Father today as you enter His presence? What will be the object of your fast, so that you may feast on His eternal love? As you look forward to standing today in His holy presence, are you also looking across the horizon to the explosive years yet to come, eagerly waiting, and expecting great things from your God as you face the future boldly with Him? If this is your soul's desire, then God will touch your tender heart as we come to that great theme and grand finale.

But all sinners will be destroyed; the future of the wicked will be cut off.

PSALM 37:38

All the rich of the earth will feast and worship; all who go down to the dust will kneel before him—those who cannot keep themselves alive. Posterity will serve him; future generations will be told about the Lord.

PSALM 22:29–30

CHAPTER TEN

Facing the Future Boldly with God

IF THE ENTIRE WORLD'S population were condensed to a small village of only one hundred people, what kind of a community do you think we'd be looking at? Would it be an enjoyable, exciting, happy place to live, where people got along because of their similarities and their access to the privileges of life? Or would it be a difficult, perhaps even a depressing, living environment because of the chasm of inequality that existed between its people? What would be the racial components of such a spot? How many men would live there? How many women? Who would be the primary owners of the real estate, the banks, and the houses? What would be the general quality of life of this village's citizens? Based on today's real world statistics, these questions have been answered by compressing the population of planet earth into just such a village of one hundred people, with these results:

- 57 would be Asian
- 8 would be African
- 51 would be female
- 21 would be European
- 14 would be from the Western Hemisphere
- 49 would be male
- 30 would be white

- 50 percent of the wealth would reside in the hands of six people
- 70 would be unable to read
- 50 would be suffering from malnutrition
- 80 would be struggling to survive in substandard housing
- One would be near death
- One would be giving birth
- One would have a college education
- No one would own a computer

Where do we fit into this compressed, global village? Would we be the leaders of the community? Own property? Would we live well, or might we find ourselves scarcely making it, just hanging on, almost over the edge of poverty and starvation? Would our race be in the majority, or in the minority? Would we be envied for our financial status and perhaps even feel defensive about our wealth—maybe even a little afraid others might want what we possessed? How many great novels, theological treatises, and weekly magazines would we have stored in our libraries—that is, if we had the ability to afford them, and, of course, be able to read? Would we be in robust health, or would we and our families be chronically ill? Would it be a village we'd enjoy living in, a model place to raise our families, or would the widespread pain, sorrow, and lack of hope in the eyes of our fellow citizens cause us to weep for their tortured bodies and their lost, eternal souls?

These are all legitimate questions, because this is the village in which we live. Welcome to the real world on the eve of the twenty-first century.

When I realize the status I would enjoy in this compressed global village, I feel a pain in my heart, because I would immediately have such a great advantage over most of my fellow villagers. I would be regarded as a person of tremendous privilege, of more than ample means, basking in good health and glowing opportunities for personal growth, while most of my neighbors would have virtually nothing of this world's goods, agonizing with terrible, life-threatening diseases, with little or no opportunity to get ahead and, quite possibly, because of their malnourished condition, not have the physical strength or mental acuity even to be able to *hear* the Good News of Jesus Christ.

How will the poor, the desperate, and the physically and spiritually dying of our world—a world that includes the United States—ever find the freedom to face the future boldly with God?

THE VILLAGE IS HERE

The troubling thing for me to grasp is that I already *live* in this village, and so do you. Has the truth of this fact hit you yet? We already live there! So we must ask ourselves some tough questions. How will the poor, the desperate, and the physically and spiritually dying of our world—a world that includes the United States—ever find the freedom to face the future boldly with God? What will it take for the disenfranchised to know the Truth, and to have that Truth liberate them once and for all from the chains that bind them—chains of hunger, superstition, and dying religions that create nothing but fear, and that provide no hope for the present *or* the future?

Will it be enough for us to pray an occasional prayer for those who suffer? Or shall we simply take an offering during a special Sunday service and designate it to help meet their needs? Or perhaps we should check out books from the library or surf the Internet to access the raw statistical data which will inform us just how bad their condition *really* is? Is this enough? Is this all we need to do, especially when we have serious challenges of our own—our own spiritual hunger, along with the normal difficulties *we* face in our daily lives like just paying our bills, keeping our jobs, and struggling to maintain a high standard of morality in our homes so that our children will know the difference between what is right and wrong in a society that has blurred the distinction?

IT'S NOT EITHER . . . OR

Tough choices during tough times. But I would submit that it does not—must not—be an *either . . . or* situation. We must do both: reach out to a world in need, as well as take care of business at home. The apostle Paul addressed this issue when he wrote to his son in the faith, Timothy: "If anyone does not provide for his relatives, and especially for his immediate family, he has denied the faith and is worse than an unbeliever (1 Timothy 5:8). And the only way I know for us to maintain the courage, strength, and tenacity to grasp these challenges, and to make any significant progress on either front, is to ask God to give us His wisdom and insight to walk through His gateway to supernatural power. We must live a life of humbling ourselves in fasting and prayer to see the world as God sees it: suffering, dying, agonizing, and without hope.

✳ **Let my heart be broken with the things that break the heart of God.**

If we attempt to wade into the uncharted waters of our future in our own limited strength, we will have no enduring effect on the culture in which we live or in the world that surrounds us and increasingly encroaches on us. If we only shed a few tears, give a few dollars, read a few articles, and pray a few perfunctory prayers, our influence will be the same as taking a teaspoon to the ocean with an attempt to drain it dry. In the haunting words of Bob Pierce, founder of World Vision, we too must say, "Let my heart be broken with the things that break the heart of God."

When will our spirits be crushed by the cruelty we see on the television news? When will we call racism what it is, both at home and abroad? When will we humble ourselves in repentant fasting and prayer before God, saying, *"Father, I don't know what to do, and I know I can't do it all. Please, in Your mercy, make me understand what You want me to be, and what You want me to do as humanity faces this uncertain future—so many face it without You."*

ARE WE PREACHING TO THE CHOIR?

This is the prayer that will bring us closer to God's heart, even as we do our part as members of the Body of Christ to bring closure to the Great Commission that still demands we go into *all* the world, preaching, teaching, loving, baptizing, and being God's servants to those who don't know the Savior. Only with this attitude can we—dare we—face the future boldly with God. Anything less will be feeble attempts to engage in shopworn, standard business procedures which will not win the day, will not bring revival to our individual hearts, to our churches, to our nation, or to our world.

☀ **Some 90 percent of all evangelistic efforts are aimed at people within the Christian world, 95 percent of all Christian activity is for the benefit of Christians, and 99 percent of all Christian publishing and writing addresses topics of interest only to Christians.**

Sharing the Good News is all about Christians being in serious contact with those who don't know the Savior. If there's no such contact, then there's no mission going on. Well-known missions researcher David Barrett has compared the amount of contact between these two groups today and five centuries ago. He estimated that in the last decade of the 1400s only 19 percent of the world's population was Christian. Since all but 7 percent of these believers were concentrated in Europe, only 2 percent of the world's non-Christians had any contact with Christianity. Due to advances in mass communications and transportation, he reminds us, there is a great deal more contact today. Barrett says that 44 percent of the world's population has some knowledge of Christianity through contact with the 33 percent of the world's people who are Christians. Although that leaves only 23 percent of the world's population completely untouched by Christianity, Barrett emphasized that that still means 1.2 billion people have absolutely no knowledge of the gospel. Some 90 percent of all evangelistic efforts are aimed at people within the Christian world, 95 percent of all Christian activity is for the benefit of Christians, and 99 percent of all Christian publishing and writing addresses topics of interest only to Christians.[1]

UNNOTICED OPPORTUNITIES

Is revival needed in our land? In our world? How long will we continue to lull ourselves to sleep by seeking and enjoying the creature benefits of upward mobility, rather than following Christ's example of suffering and sacrifice? The urban poor, both at home and around the world, afflicted as they are with mounting disease, homelessness, soaring crime rates, and addictions to everything from sex to drugs, have never been more open to the liberating Good News of Jesus Christ. Yet this enormous opportunity has gone largely unnoticed, and even studiously avoided, by vast numbers of us who say we are followers of Jesus Christ.

The crying need is for people who are willing to go into the cities, live among the hurting multitudes, and lead them into a living and growing relationship with Jesus Christ. In centuries past, urban warriors like William Booth and George Mueller gave up the comforts of middle-class life in order to challenge the forces of hell in the cities of Britain. Today we need men and women who will make the same kinds of sacrifices to gather in the harvest He has prepared.

PAYING THE PRICE

Who will be that man? Who will be that woman? Will it be you? Will it be me? How will we know if God has put His divine hand on us to be part of this massive outpouring of His Spirit in our time? Again, I say the only way I know that we'll be quiet and attentive enough to hear God's voice is through the godly disciplines of fasting and prayer. Only when we experience the depth of God and His love will we be able to rise to newness of life. But it will be necessary to pay the price, just as we will always pay a price for something that is lasting and worthwhile. Paying the price will cost us some conveniences.

To fast means to deny ourselves what is common, normal, and necessary—food—for a period of time so that our minds will become sharp, our hearts softened, and our spirits receptive to what God has to say to us. God promises to fill the void that the absence of food creates; He will pour out His blessings and sate us in a way that food neither can nor will. Without this intentional, heightened spiritual focus that comes from humbling ourselves in God's presence, we will be doomed to face the future timidly, defensively, without power, and without serious motivation. But when we have been in the presence of almighty God, and have taken our direction from His heart, we will have the wherewithal, the strength, the desire, the courage, and the confidence to face the future boldly, without fear, and without compromise.

THE REWARDS OF JOURNALING

When God calls you to fast, one of the most helpful outcomes will be what you record in your daily journals. They will be filled with intimate conversations between you and God—dialogs with your heavenly Father you have never had before. Your journals will contain Scripture, promises you make to God, and reminders of God's promises to you, praise statements, and answers to your most desperate prayers. My own fasting journals chronicle my struggling pilgrimage of desperately wanting to know the God of Moses and Abraham, Isaac, and Jacob—servants who could face *their* futures boldly because they had been with their Creator on holy ground. Page after page of my journals show my weakness and lack of fortitude as I found myself getting closer to God's righteousness and power. I wrote honestly my every thought, my every motive, my hurts, my joys, my tears, and my desires. Over a period of several fasts, I wrote the following as an exercise of my spiritual worship:

I pray and fast at this time for the purpose of humbling myself before You, to be in continual touch with You, to experience the immediacy of Your presence, and to receive the authority of Jesus in my life. As a minister of the Lord, may I stand in the gap for my nation and God. May the Holy Spirit be my power and my authority. May my heart be broken as I give it to You. May God withhold His judgment and pour out His Spirit on all mankind.

I pray today that I will be Your man. Not man's man, not almighty man, but God's man. I pray I will do all and be all God wants me to be and do. May the Lord be God upon me today. May my soul pant for Thee, my God. May I thirst for You, O my Living God. Even as I fast from food, may I have an appetite to be with You, and allow You to nourish me with Yourself.

Anoint me with the oil of Jesus' joy. O God, speak to me. In Jesus' name, speak to me. Be glorified in me. I need Your Word. My trust is in You, O God. I pray for God to do more in a moment today than I could ever do in a lifetime. O God, give me Your passion and Your heart. May I simply be Your representative today and every day.

To You alone be the praise for guiding and strengthening me during this forty-day fast. O God, I pray for the hand of my God to be upon me. I praise You for the affirmation of James 4:10, "Humble yourselves in the presence of the Lord, and He will exalt you." O God, You have given a "greater grace" to those who humble themselves before Your holy face.

Fill me with the fire of the Spirit and the joy of the Lord. I ask that Your power be upon me. Let me be an instrument of God to see people released from physical, emotional, and spiritual bondage, both at home and throughout the world. Thank You God for these forty days. I give them—and all that comes out of them—to the glory of Jesus. May this be only the beginning of a new life and walk with You.

What will your journal record about your time with God as you approach His presence in fasting and prayer? I don't know. But I promise you that when you let your heart be open to the heart of our Father, whatever you write will be a true reflection of your future direction as a child of the King. Because you have been in His holy presence, you will never again feel alone. You will never again wonder if *God is really alive.* You will never again entertain the thought that your heavenly Father may be a silent God, removed from your personal concerns and challenges. These will be thoughts from your distant past because you have been in the presence of the King. When all else fails, and when all *others* fail you, He alone will be your guiding light.

A STAR TO GUIDE US

The artist had crafted a masterpiece—an oil painting of a solitary figure rowing a boat across a sea at night. In the far distance he had painted a solitary star, shining alone, but with great brilliance. Those who viewed the painting could get but one impression: If the person in the rowboat ever lost contact with that lonely star in the sky, he would be lost. Doomed. Without hope of finding his way. The star was the rower's only source of direction. He had no map. No artificial light. It was the star alone that guided him, illumination from afar that would assure him of making it to his destination. He didn't focus his attention on the boat or his oars or even the tumultuous waves that lay ahead. The rower fixed his eyes on the star. His only light and only hope.

What that painting should say to us is that when we feel we're all alone, rowing across our own sea of darkness and despair, our star—our heavenly Father—shines in His heavens as our constant and abiding light. But if we lose sight of the light of Jesus, we will be utterly lost. He's our star—our singular reason to face the future boldly with confidence, courage, and hope. He's our beacon when the other nonlights of the world grow dim. An unknown poet has written,

> *Jesus, be a guiding star before me.*
> *Be a soothing wake behind me.*
> *Be a rolling path below me.*
> *Be a flaming hope within me.*
> *Be all these things—now and forever.*

But if we lose sight of the light of Jesus, we will be utterly lost. He's our star—our singular reason to face the future boldly with confidence, courage, and hope.

NO GIMMICKS, NO HYPE

Jesus was my guiding star on a recent ministry trip to India— land of one billion people, second only in population to China, and yet only one-third of the land mass of the United States. As our plane was about to land in Bombay, my prayer was simply "Jesus, help me see, feel, and hear what you experience in Your Father's heart as *You* look into the faces I am about to meet."

It was my first trip to India, but I had a strong sense of what I was about to experience. I knew I would see human pain in monumental proportions, but I didn't want to be so thrown off by the physical poverty and human misery that I would fail to see deep into their souls. So I prayed, "Lord, help me to see the crying needs of these men and women, but may I see beyond the physical to the spiritual urgency of the people You have created and who live in this land."

The first night I observed that forty thousand people sat quietly on the ground, eager, attentive, and open to hearing God's Word. That night we all saw an extreme movement of the Spirit of God. People who had never once heard the gospel said yes to the Savior. Friends back home were praying and fasting that we would see a mighty stirring of the Spirit of God in that place. Their prayers were answered.

The next night, I spoke to more than seventy-five thousand spiritually hungry men and women, who wanted to hear God's Word. My host, Dr. K. A. Paul, an Indian evangelist, considered by many to be the Billy Graham of India, gave the main message as those thousands of Indians sat motionless in the presence of a holy God as His messengers spoke of their need for a Savior and Lord. Many wonder why Dr. Paul is enjoying such an outpouring of God's blessing as he ministers to his people. I know that it's because he spends time with his God in fasting and prayer.

I have never seen such a stream of humanity. They stood, and they stood, and when it was over, more than 50,000 had asked Jesus Christ to come into their lives.

There were no gimmicks, no hype, no bells, and no whistles. In their physical and spiritual poverty, they streamed into that arena looking for something their own religion has never been able to offer them—peace for today and hope for their future. Dr. Paul already knew what lay ahead for many of those who had come that evening. He himself had been beaten, kidnapped, and left for dead because he had preached the blood of Jesus without fear or compromise. As he shared his experiences with me, I couldn't help but think of how he had suffered for his faith without complaint. I also wondered if we at home would be willing to pay such a price. When it came time to invite people to step forward to make a personal commitment to Jesus Christ, Dr. Paul made it clear what he wanted the people to do, if God had called them to present themselves before Him. In fact, he even tried to talk them *out* of coming, fearing they might not understand that taking a stand for Jesus could cost them their lives. But they would hear nothing of his disclaimers or attempts to persuade them to stay seated, not even after he spent another ten minutes telling them what might happen to them if they put their faith and trust in the Savior.

WILLING TO PAY THE PRICE

Then, it was as if heaven opened. I could hardly believe it. They stood up in the back, on the sides, and in the front. I have never seen such a stream of humanity. They stood, and they stood, and when it was over, more than fifty thousand people had asked Jesus Christ to come into their lives, to give them hope, to make them whole, and to provide them with a certain future. They were willing to pay the price, ready to take their stand, no matter what the cost.

In that fresh, new setting, I caught their excitement of the gospel as they were hearing it for the first time. I had known the

Christian faith since I was a child. I knew the right answers long before I'd bothered to ask the questions. Could it be that I had somehow become overly comfortable with my knowledge of the gospel? Had I just been coasting along in my ministry, so familiar with God that I had taken Him for granted? I searched my own soul as I watched them respond by the thousands. I asked God to keep breaking my heart with the things that broke His own heart.

Later, with my spirit moved beyond my ability to describe it adequately, God also gave me the opportunity to address twelve hundred Indian pastors. Most were from eighteen to twenty-three years of age. They had no theological degrees, and little, if any, Bible school training, but in their eyes I saw sacrifice. I saw Jesus. I saw compassion for the people with whom they would soon be sharing God's Good News. I was told that many of those pastors would suffer such persecution that they would surely be killed. Many of their fellow pastors had already been tortured, and even chopped into pieces, because of their faith in Jesus. I left India enriched because of the work of grace God had done in my heart.

THE REASON WE MUST WAKE UP THROUGH
PRAYER AND FASTING

Earlier in this chapter we talked about the desperate condition of our lost and dying world. Today, there is a band of countries that fall into what missiologists call the "10/40 Window." The top 50 percent of the world's least evangelized cities are located in this area. If you take a world map and look between 10 degrees north to 40 degrees north of the equator, you will discover this "10/40 Window" with 66 countries of the world that comprise approximately 4.1 billion people. Out of these 4.1 billion people, there may be upwards to 3 billion people who have never heard the name of Jesus. India is one of those countries. In my visit to that nation and to the "10/40 Window," God made it clear to me what we must do in America.

We must wake up, pray, and fast in our own nation. I'm more convinced than ever that we will not see revival in the church of America until we deal with our sin of not taking the gospel to the unreached peoples of the world. How dare we be so presumptuous as to expect God to visit the American church if we don't demonstrate a strong, serious commitment to finding *the heart of God*, which is to take the Good News of Jesus Christ to those who have not yet heard.

The American church must make an intentional commitment to bringing closure to the Great Commission in our generation. We must do this by shaking ourselves from our lazy slumber and by fasting and praying. The word "nations," found in Matthew 28:19–20, means *subcultures,* not necessarily *countries* as we know the world today. The challenge and mission of the American church must be to take the gospel to every one of these subcultures in our world. The task is enormous, and our spiritual nerve must be ready for the task. But praise God, this mission is already underway. We're doing it through modern technology, and because God is raising up thousands of dedicated Christians throughout the world who are preaching the gospel in places where it has never been proclaimed at any time in history! This is how God is bringing closure to the Great Commission. This is the exciting time Jesus spoke of in Matthew 24:14, "And this gospel of the kingdom will be preached in the whole world as a testimony to all nations, and then the end will come."

❋ **The American church must make an intentional commitment to bringing closure to the Great Commission in our generation, and we must do this by shaking ourselves from our lazy slumber and by fasting and praying.**

We are seeing it with our own eyes! History is winding down. But while God's work is vibrant and alive in so many places, we as a nation are still fast asleep, snoring our way through what should be the most exciting time of our lives. It is time for America to wake up. We must repent of our sin of selfishness, of spending our time and most of our resources on our own selfish pleasures. We must become increasingly active in taking the gospel of Jesus Christ to *all* unreached subcultures, not only here in desperately needy America, and not only in the "10/40 Window," but across the world.

FIGHTING ON THE RIGHT SIDE

As I flew back to the United States, my heart was *satisfied*—a word from the Latin which means to be filled. Sated. I was satisfied that thousands had given their hearts to Jesus, satisfied that God had shown me how so many new believers were ready to face the future boldly with God. The writer, G. K. Chesterton, once said that "In the end it will not matter to us whether we wrote well or ill; whether we fought with flails or reeds. It will matter to us greatly on what side we fought." Only then will we have known satisfaction. I knew Dr. Paul and I had fought on the right side during those few days of ministry in India. God had satisfied our hearts, while at the same time He had created enormous dissatisfaction in our spirits with the awareness of the great work that still needs to be done.

WHEN GOD ACTS . . .

More than six hundred years before Christ was born, the prophet Isaiah predicted that Christ's work of service on the cross would result in His satisfaction at the resurrection. Isaiah wrote, "After the suffering of his soul, he will see the light and be satisfied; by his knowledge my righteous servant will justify many, and he will bear their iniquities" (53:11). Again, that word *satisfied.* Filled to overflowing. Complete. What can we learn from Christ's example? Certainly we learn that service isn't going to be easy. There *will* be suffering of our souls. Service will not be convenient. For some, it will mean pain, possibly even death. But if God directs us and gives us His strength, then our service will be satisfying. Martin Lloyd-Jones wrote, "When God acts, He can do more in a minute than man with his organizing can do in fifty years." I would add, "or in a lifetime!"

When God calls us to fast and pray, we are connected with the only true source of supernatural power, and we are linked to a God who cleanses our hearts and purifies our spirits. As he makes us clean, He removes the dissonance and static that have short-circuited our communion with God. As we fast and pray, we sharpen our focus as God lifts our spirits. When we choose not to be sated—satisfied—with physical food during our fast, our heavenly Father satisfies us with the delight of His presence. At first it is all so new, so unexpected. Then He takes hold of our eager hearts and speaks as we've never heard Him before. Once connected with our almighty, omnipotent heavenly Father, we begin to receive His supernatural power to fight an unnatural war—not a battle whose arsenal is filled with physical weapons of destruction, but a warfare of the spirit, of unseen powers and threats, a war we are destined to win.

CLEANSED BY HIS HOLY PRESENCE

What purifies our hearts in the presence of God? It is repentance and the confession of our estrangement from the One who made us, loves us, and wants to dwell in us. We are purified by making restitution with those who have offended us or whom we have offended. We are made clean by meditating on God's holy Word and applying what we learn in God's presence to the world in which we live. We are purified by the time we spend in prayer as we bring our deepest needs, our fondest dreams, and greatest hopes to the feet of Jesus. Our spiritual bones become strong, and our spiritual arteries, designed by our Creator to flow with love and kindness, become unclogged. We begin to see life as God intended for us to live it. We suddenly realize it's not the physical food but the spiritual nourishment that we receive from our Lord that gives us our power, determination, courage, and hope.

THE KEY TO GREATNESS

Who is this mighty God? God, through His Son Jesus, is the prophet of the one who's humble, not the person who is proud. He proclaims that the first will be last, that the weak are the strong, and that the foolish are wise. He says that the poor and lowly, not the proud, possess the kingdom of heaven. He declares that greatness in His sight will come only through service to Him. In Matthew 20:25–28, we read:

> Jesus called them together and said, "You know that the rulers of the Gentiles lord it over them, and their high officials exercise authority over them. Not so with you. Instead, whoever wants to become great among you must be your servant, and whoever wants to be first must be your slave—

just as the Son of Man did not come to be served, but to serve, and to give his life as a ransom for many."

✳ **Fasting and prayer do not come naturally. We will have to reorder our priorities, reschedule our commitments, and revise our minuscule, man-made plans to make the time to be in the presence of the Lord.**

The key to greatness in the Kingdom of God is neither power nor position. Greatness is to be conformed to the image of Jesus Christ. If we want to identify with Jesus in His glory, we must also identify with him in His humility. A true servant looks for legitimate needs to meet, whether at home or across the ocean, ministering to others with joy and understanding. But for us to stay the course, to know the supernatural power of God, and to be able to face the future boldly and with confidence, demands that we be alert to the vehicles that give us immediate access to enormous power—the disciplines of prayer and fasting. And they are disciplines. Fasting and prayer do not come naturally. We will have to reorder our priorities, reschedule our commitments, and revise our minuscule, man-made plans to make the time to be in the presence of the Lord. That is what these Old Testament saints did as they took God seriously in their lives.

- Abraham rose early to stand before the Lord. (Genesis 19:27)

- Jacob rose early to worship the Lord. (Genesis 28:18)

- Hannah and Elkanah rose early to worship God. (1 Samuel 1:9)

- Moses rose up early to give God's message to Pharaoh. (Exodus 8:20)

- Joshua rose up early to capture Jericho. (Joshua 6:12)
- Gideon rose up early to examine the fleece. (Judges 6:38)

What are we willing to do to come into His holy presence? Are we willing . . .

- to close the book of complaints and open the book of God's praise?

- to ignore what we feel life owes us and think more about what we owe others?

- to stop looking for friendship and start being a friend?

- to be content with the material things God has already given us and stop fretting about the things we have not?

- to enjoy God's simple blessings and stop striving for the artificial pleasures of the day?

- to cease looking for someone to help us and begin devoting ourselves to a lifetime of service in helping others come to know our Savior?

- to see a spiritual awakening of a world, a nation, a community, and a church, *starting in our hearts*, and through fasting and prayer enter God's gateway to supernatural power for the intense spiritual warfare that is yet ahead?

You may say, "But I'm just one person, only a flickering candle in a windy world that doesn't give its allegiance to Jesus. What can I do when I feel so alone, wondering if God can use me and my limited capacities?"

If you feel you're in the minority in your walk with God, you have suddenly put yourself in good biblical company:

- When **Noah** was building the ark, he was very much in the minority—but he followed his Creator, and God blessed Noah and his family.

- When **Joseph** was sold into Egypt by his brothers, he was in the minority, and even though his brothers meant it for evil, God meant it for good.

- When **Gideon** and his three hundred followers, with their broken pitchers and lamps, put the Midianites to flight, they were in the minority, but the battle was won and God was honored.

- When **Elijah** prayed down fire from heaven and put the prophets of Baal to shame, he was in the minority, but he won the day.

- When **David**, ridiculed by his brothers, went out to meet the giant Goliath, in size and influence young David was in a decided minority, but God ruled that day, and the enemy was defeated.

- When **Jesus** was crucified by Roman soldiers, by all appearances He seemed to be in a conspicuous minority, but He didn't stay on the cross, nor did He remain in the tomb. He arose, and He lives today for you, for me, and for a world waiting to have a reason to face the future with boldness and courage. With God as the source of our power, we will never be in the minority, and we will never be alone.

Do we have our hearts set on God? Do we want to elevate our relationships with our Creator to new levels? Have we had enough of business-as-usual religion, playing church, attending meetings that are meaningless, and seeing no real influence in our witness on the lives of others? If you are compelled to say yes, then I hope you are persuaded to be attentive to the call of God for your life. He may have been calling you all the time, but the noise of life and the distractions of daily living may have kept that call from falling on your ears. This may be the moment you say with Job, "Teach me, and I will be quiet; show me where I have been wrong" (Job 6:24). Or to pray with the psalmist, "Be still before the LORD and wait patiently for him" (Psalm 37:7).

For it's only in silence and our humble prayers that we will ever know God's best for our lives. It's my earnest prayer that you will have the courage to step into His presence as your first step to facing the future boldly with your loving, almighty God. If that is your decision, I encourage you use the following pages as your guide. I'm praying for you and want God's best for you in all the exciting days that lie ahead. Our prayed-for revival *will* come, because we desperately need a fresh touch from God. Whether we drift from God, become distracted by competing interests, or simply become overwhelmed by the struggles of life, we need to reconnect with our heavenly Father. As we humble ourselves *individually* to pray and fast, an awakening will also come to our churches, our nation and to our world, but it will only come to others when it first comes to us. I close these pages with a message that is as fresh today as it was the day our Lord and Savior gave it to those who had ears to hear:

> When you fast, do not look somber as the hypocrites do, for they disfigure their faces to show men they are fasting. I tell you the truth, they have received their reward in full. But when you fast, put oil on your head and wash your face, so that it will not be obvious to men that you are fasting, but only to your Father, who is unseen; and your Father, who sees what is done in secret, will reward you. Do not store up

for yourselves treasures on earth, where moth and rust destroy, and where thieves break in and steal. But store up for yourselves treasures in heaven, where moth and rust do not destroy, and where thieves do not break in and steal. For where your treasure is, there your heart will be also.

—Matthew 6:16–21

A PRACTICAL GUIDE

Fasting and Prayer as Your Spiritual Worship

THE DISCIPLINES OF PRAYER AND FASTING are not re-duced to a formula or a hoop that we are to jump through as if we are in a kind of spiritual circus. Nor are they physical tests or exercises in mental discipline. True prayer and fasting are attitudes of the heart and cries of the soul. God's Word has a strong rebuke for those who fast for the wrong reasons or in an improper manner. I have never seen God respond favorably to prayer and/or fasting based on false pretenses or impure motives.

Improper Reasons/Motives

Prayer and fasting are improper when a person seeks . . .
- to fulfill selfish desires and ambitions.
- to attempt to manipulate God.
- to elevate one's status or personal agenda.
- to promote false piety, legalism, or religious duty.

Improper Manner

Prayer and fasting are improper when they . . .
- draw attention to personal glorification.
- are attempted without sufficient seriousness and respect.
- are conducted while intentionally continuing in sin.
- are conducted while continuing to pursue selfish desires in pleasure and business.

- are conducted while harboring improper, ungodly attitudes.
- are conducted while promoting or continuing injustice, oppression, or impropriety.
- are conducted without drawing aside daily and dedicating ample time for sincere seeking, quiet communion, and devoted prayer with God.

GOD-HONORING FAST

The Bible is filled with references to the prayers and fasting of His people. In Matthew 6, Jesus placed fasting on the same level as praying and giving. He said, "When you fast, when you pray, and when you give." I wonder why Christians today and churches in our generation don't place fasting on the same level as praying and giving? Jesus, by His example and His teaching, demonstrates that prayer and fasting are important and integral ingredients in the lives of His followers. One purpose of prayer and fasting is to bring our hearts to a place of being filled with a sacrificial love that results in godly attitudes in our lives. True fasting will draw us closer to God and His purposes.

I can't explain why God has chosen prayer and fasting as the gateway to supernatural power. One thing I do know: Scripture, prayer, and fasting are the ways believers humble themselves in the sight of the Lord. When we humble ourselves, He promises to exalt and lift us up at the appointed time (1 Peter 5:6; James 4:10). God also indicates that He will resist the proud, but will give grace to the humble (James 4:6). Again, 2 Chronicles 7:14 indicates the importance of humbling ourselves before God.

Fasting brings a sharp focus to the dramatic difference between our physical and spiritual natures. Eating is one of the most fundamental things we do as physical beings. One of the most natural desires is for food. Without proper nourishment we die. By exercising our wills and depriving ourselves of food for spiritual purposes, we acknowledge our spiritual natures and honor our Creator-Father. When we deny the natural for the purpose of calling upon God to do the supernatural, He will enable and empower us to experience the supernatural. Through fasting, we confirm the words uttered by Jesus in the face of temptation during His forty day fast, "Man does not live by bread alone, but by every Word that proceeds from the mouth of God" (Matthew 4:4). Through prayer and fasting we forsake our own physical needs and the creature comforts of this world and call upon God as the Originator, Giver, Source, and Sustainer of all life, especially our own. We exalt Him as our hope and salvation. True spiritual fasting will results in submission and devotion to God.

GOD BLESSES US WHEN OUR FASTS . . .

- focus on Him and honor Him. (Although you will receive spiritual blessings, these are not proper motives for fasting.)
- have spiritual purposes. (Although you may realize certain physical benefits, these are not proper motives for spiritual fasting, e.g. for weight-loss purposes.)
- cause individuals to humble themselves and submit to the authority of God and His Word.
- cause individuals to acknowledge and repent of sin.
- deprive our natural desires and lusts to focus on the spiritual.

A PRACTICAL GUIDE

Even when we honor God by praying and fasting, this does not mean that our heavenly Father will grant everything on our wish-and-whim list. God will only work and bless in ways that are consistent and in harmony with His will and purpose. One of the primary functions of prayer and fasting is to help us discover what His ordained purposes and will are for our lives.

I have included some practical helps and hints that are rooted in my own experience—guidelines that I follow as I fast and pray.

Spiritual Suggestions

- If God does not call you to fast, don't fast! Most people don't have a call to fast possibly because they're not totally open to God's leadership, have not been taught the biblical foundation for fasting, or are caught up in other types of sin that interfere.

- Determine in advance the length of the fast God is calling you to undertake.

- If God calls you to a fast, He has specific reasons and purposes in mind. Before you fast, determine the purposes of your fast and write them down, e.g. "Lord, I am fasting for the spiritual purposes of: (1) spiritual revival and awakening in the church of America, (2) spiritual revival and awakening in my own local church, and (3) spiritual revival and awakening in my own personal life. Under each of these major headings there could be several subpoints about what you are trusting God for in each of these areas.

- Identify, confess, and repent of all revealed sin before and during your fast. Continue to ask the Holy Spirit to search your heart and reveal any concealed areas where you may feel separated from God. Unconfessed sin and disobedience will hinder your prayer and fasting.

- Be sensitive to the Holy Spirit's prompting in all areas of your life, since God will often require you to seek reconciliation or restoration in broken relationships.

- Pray fervently and continually.

- Absorb large quantities of Scripture into your life through hearing, reading, studying, memorizing, and meditating on God's Word. Ask God to reveal what He wants you to read and study in His Word.

- Always reserve time to be still and quiet before the Lord.

- Keep a journal of your purposes for the fast. A limited journal has been provided beginning on page 217. This should contain specific prayer requests, written prayers, devotional thoughts, and spiritual insights you are gaining during your fast. For example, I handwrite many of my prayers to God. I also document whatever I feel God is teaching me, even though they may seem insignificant at the time. I include the specific day and time in the journal entry. These daily writings have been a consistent source of encouragement, strength, and insight long after the fast has ended, reminding me, often months later, of God's direction and calling for my life.

- Skipping meals alone will not result in a meaningful fast! You must *set aside time* to pray and seek spiritual insight. Dedicate at least as much time as you would normally spend in food preparation and eating for prayer and the study of God's Word.

- Consider praying audibly in a kneeling position. At times, try getting on your face before God. This may help foster an attitude of humility in prayer and keep you focused on your purposes.

- Praise God verbally and in song for who He is and what He has done: Worship Him.

- Use scriptural prayers during some of your prayer time.

- Ask God with whom, when, and how you may want to share your fasting experience when it has come to an end. If God so allows it, your testimony can challenge, inspire, and help increase the faith of others. Always give God the glory for what He has done in your life.

Physical Suggestions

- As a precautionary measure, check with your doctor before beginning your first fast.

- Eat mainly raw foods and drink plenty of water for a few meals before you begin your fast.

- Decrease the size and frequency of meals before beginning your fast, especially a prolonged fast.

- Determine in advance what kind of fast you will undertake, e.g. total abstinence, water only, water and juice, etc. I recommend water-and-juice fasts. They help you accomplish the spiritual and physical purposes of the fast, while at the same time, they help you to maintain your energy level and your health.

- Avoid chewing gum during the fast. Chewing activates the digestive processes.

- Days *two through four* of the fast are often the most challenging.

- When drinking juice on a fast, nonsweetened and nonacidic

juices seem best. Tomato and orange juice are hard on the stomach, unless greatly diluted.

- Most of my juice was prepared at home. Since I knew I would be entering a prolonged fast, one of the purchases I made was a professional juicer.

- If you (a) undertake a water-only fast, (b) plan an extended fast, (c) have a medical condition, or (d) are taking medication, you should consult a medical doctor familiar with fasting before you begin your fast.

- Consult other resources on fasting.

- You may need to restrict some of your physical activity during the fast, especially rigorous exercise.

- Sudden movements, especially standing up quickly, may cause temporary dizziness or lightheadedness.

- Expect some physical, mental and, perhaps, even some emotional discomfort. Headaches, sleeplessness, and irritability often accompany a fast, but don't allow the fast to become an excuse for improper actions and attitudes.

- You will likely experience some weight loss during a fast, but the weight usually returns quickly once the fast is broken.

- It's important always to consider the feelings of others, particularly family members, when planning a fast. For example, to plan a fast during a holiday or a family reunion could unnecessarily offend others or draw attention to yourself. Ask God for *the right time* to conduct your fast.

- Some people, even those with good intentions, may try to keep you from fasting; others may encourage you to end your fast before the appointed time. You should anticipate this and be prepared with a kind, yet resolved, response.

- End the fast, especially an extended one, gradually. After my prolonged fasts, I eat only soft foods for at least a couple of days (baked potato, soup, yogurt, etc.). I begin with small portions and gradually increase my intake. I then move to other foods that are more easily digested. I often wait five or more days before returning to a full meal. Returning to normal eating patterns too quickly after a fast can cause serious medical problems, and may also minimize some of the physical benefits of the fast.

ANSWERS TO SOME OF THE MOST COMMONLY ASKED QUESTIONS

Q: *How do you know if you're called to a fast?*

A: The fasts God has called me to have been as clear and specific as anything He has ever asked me to do in my life. In all cases, the deep burden and sincere conviction I experienced were unmistakably from God. Usually, if confusion prevails regarding the fast, it is not God's timing to draw aside. The Lord will make it clear if He wants you to fast, especially for a prolonged period of time.

Q: *During your extended fasts, what type and quantities of liquid did you consume?*

A: During my extended fasts, the first couple of days I consumed only water. At the conclusion of the second day or at the beginning of the third day, I began drinking various kinds of juices that have been prepared at home in a professional juicer.

My wife would prepare these juices from fresh fruit and vegetables. I most enjoyed juices made from watermelon, cantaloupe, grape, pineapple, and grapefruit. Watermelon juice was particularly effective to reduce an occasional headache. Grapefruit juice helped with the cleansing effect of the fast. Typically, I would drink eight to twelve ounces of juice four times a day. I would consume water throughout the day. On some days, I would also drink some Gatorade™ (because it was refreshing, provided variety, and also helped ease an occasional headache).

Q: *What are some of the biggest challenges you have faced during your fasts?*

A: Physically, my greatest challenges have come between the second and fourth days. On the first day, because my body was accustomed to caffeine and generous portions of food, the sudden withdrawal caused me to have some major headaches. Later in the fast, my body began to feel great. I did not experience any real physical hunger. I had adequate energy and actually felt better than normal, especially after the tenth or fourteenth day.

Although I was not physically hungry after day four or five, I would often face some mental challenges. It can be intimidating and discouraging to focus on how many days remain in your designated fast, especially early in the fast. You've heard the old question, "How do you eat an elephant? *One bite at a time.*" Similarly, "How can you fast for forty days? *By fasting one day at a time.*" It can be a torturous mental battle to count and anticipate that you have twenty or thirty more days to go in your fast. Instead, I remained focused on one day at a time.

Q: *How does a fast affect your bodily functions?*

A: Fasting cleanses your body. You have to visit the facilities more often than normal. You may experience bad breath or some unusual body odor as the body is freed up to release toxins that have built up in your system.

Q: *Have you ever failed in a fast? What should someone do if he or she fails in the fast?*

A: No, I've not failed, if failure means not successfully completing the number of days that I had originally committed. I felt deeply that God had called me to the fast, and I remained confident He would enable me to accomplish that which He had asked me to do. If God has called you to a fast and you fail to start or finish, then confess this inaction, repent of it, ask God to give you another opportunity, and then wait for Him to call you to another fast.

Q: *What do you write in your spiritual journal?*

A: In both prolonged fasts, I have recorded many pages of handwritten notes to myself and to God. I will often begin by simply writing, "Dear God," and then continue to write whatever is on my heart. The prayers are usually related to the specific purposes of my fast, but I don't intentionally restrict what or for whom I pray. I also record, "God, You have spoken to me through this Scripture . . ." and then I write down the scriptural reference and the principles He has revealed to me. I always record the date and time when I am writing my journal entry. I also develop a list of things to pray for during the fast. The point is not how many pages you write, but that you record God's working in your life.

Q: *What Scriptures do you recommend for study during a fast?*

A: Each person should seek God's direction in this matter. Often, when God calls you to fast, He has already given you the passage on which to focus. Isaiah 58 and Luke 4 are good foundations upon which to build your fast. I freely mark in my study Bible, identifying key passages, phrases, or words. I also record notes on its pages. I supplement my Bible study by reading new books.

Q: *How do you handle mealtimes with your family or business associates during a fast?*

A: During the first few days, I draw aside to be alone during mealtime. After a few days, I return to sitting with the family at the table. I feel the time of sharing together is important. At that point, I am comfortable being around food. The hunger pangs are gone. The food smells good, but I'm not drawn to it. Additionally, each member of my family is aware of the fast and my reasons for it; therefore, they help to make the experience pleasant for all of us. I would restrict my lunch appointments, however, and when going out at lunchtime, I simply state, "I'm not eating today, thank you."

Q: *How do you know when to plan or schedule a fast (including length and type)?*

A: There is no simple answer to this question. I am confident that when God calls you to a fast, He will help you designate the length and type of your fast. Once I was convinced that God had called me to a forty-day fast. I prayerfully considered my calendar and looked for the best opportunity to draw aside for that purpose. The magnitude of the need may determine the length of the fast.

Q: *Have you ever been frustrated because God did not answer or lead as a result of a fast?*

A: No. One of the results of a fast is increased faith and trust in God and His sovereign will. Of course, I often have unanswered questions, but increasingly, I have less and less concern for specific answers to my concerns. I trust God to supply wisdom, guidance, and direction for my every need. True prayer and fasting result in being less concerned about having God confirm or bless *my* plans, while it increases my concern and awareness for *His* plans and purposes.

Q: *Do you believe women can and should fast in the same manner as men?*

A: Absolutely. Although there are physiological differences between men and women, prayer and fasting are not gender specific. Women can and should pray and fast. Several women in our church have gone on prolonged fasts, some for as long as forty days.

Q: *How did your family relate to you during the fast?*

A: The number one thing my family did was to pray for me. I was encouraged by their prayers, especially during our family prayer time. My two boys, Joshua and Nicholas, were great sources of inspiration to me. In addition, my wife Jeana saw her role as keeping me supplied with fresh juice and water. She faithfully ministered to me at all times.

Q: *Did you suffer any adverse effects as a result of fasting? How do you keep from allowing irritability and fatigue from affecting family relations?*

A: Although I suffered from a few headaches, I don't believe I had any adverse results from fasting. I didn't have any increased irritability. If I felt tired, I would draw aside and take a brief nap, but this only happened three or four times. My family and I approached the prolonged fasts as something of a journey. They did their best to understand the spiritual significance of the task and were tolerant, even encouraging, of my extra time alone with God and His Word. Although there were times when things around the house were a bit different because Dad was so preoccupied, they all knew this experience would be only temporary.

Q: *Whom do you tell about your fast, and when do you talk about it? Should I tell anyone about the fast or is that drawing attention to myself?*

A: I believe every person who goes on a prolonged fast should notify the people around them who will be most affected, which may be only four or five people. I tell these individuals of my intentions before I enter into the fast. My purpose is to help them understand my heart, the reasons for my fast, and to encourage them to pray for me. I am reluctant to share my fast with unbelievers. The teaching of Matthew 6:16–18 on "when you fast" is clear on how we should conduct ourselves.

Once the fast is over, I don't believe that telling people about the experience is inappropriate, especially if pure motives are maintained. Think about it this way: Moses received the Ten Commandments while fasting and praying for forty days. Imagine if he had not shared his experience with us. God gave Moses something important in his fast, and he communicated it to the people, including us these many generations later. None of the instances of prayer and fasting would appear in the Bible if fasting and its results were meant to be concealed. The key is to maintain a right spirit, a proper attitude, and motives that are pure. Much of what God reveals is a private matter; at the same time, you may help expand the faith of others by sharing with them your experience and insights, if God permits.

I would say this: During the fast do your best not to talk about it, unless you are asked and cannot avoid it. Only share about it following the fast, and only if God gives you permission.

Q: *Do you violate the principles of a God-chosen fast by publicly speaking about it?*

A: I don't believe so. Certainly, we need to hear and heed the warnings of Jesus issued in the Sermon on the Mount. His instruction does not prohibit all preaching, teaching, and discussion of prayer and fasting, but it does demand that all such communication bring glory and honor to God. If God leads you to talk about your fast with others, do it. Fasting is something *God* teaches us. Just like praying or any other principle or discipline, as we learn it, we have the privilege of sharing it. As we do, it builds our own faith and helps increase the faith of others.

Q: *How should I determine what to pray for?*

A: Before I go on a prolonged fast, I ask God for what purposes He wants me to pray and fast. For example, in both of my prolonged fasts, God directed me to pray for revival in America, in our church, and in my own life. Under each of those themes, God gave me ten to nineteen related, specific concerns or topics, e.g. the kind of awakening we need in America and how I would be involved in that revival. I prayed for each of these every day, asking the Spirit of God to teach me what to pray for, and what to trust God for during this special time in His presence.

I would begin my prayer time by confessing the sin in my life, and then enter into a time of prayer over each of the topics. I would typically end with some other specific concerns. I would then begin my study of God's Word. Usually during a prolonged fast, I would spend up to two hours each morning in prayer, reading the Word of God, and journaling. I am convinced that a person who wants a God-honoring fast will have a similar emphasis on drawing aside to pray and study God's Word.

WHAT TO EXPECT AS A RESULT OF YOUR FAST

Expect results. A properly motivated and executed fast will have an enormous impact on your life. Invariably, the primary place God seems to work is in me. As I am responsive to His lordship and leadership, I find that I must undergo some changes—changes in my thoughts, attitudes, activities, and motives. As I begin to make these changes, everything about my personal ministry and relationships change. Some are uncomfortable, challenging, and difficult. For example, as a result of one fast, I had to confront my pride and arrogance, after which I asked for forgiveness from those whom I had offended. It was important for me to take steps to change the ways I thought, acted, and reacted. Although my tendency for self-worship may resist some of the spiritual principles that God teaches, obedience to God and His Word are nonnegotiable in my life. I am convinced that obedience honors and glorifies God and will conform me to the image of Christ.

God promises to reward and bless true prayer and fasting. I

have not found a single promise that God has failed to fulfill. He honors each promise He has ever made. Here are a few of the promises God offers to those who participate in His chosen fast in Isaiah Chapter 58:6–14:

- He will set you free from self and your sinful nature. He will loosen the bonds of wickedness and undo the bands of the yoke.

- He will bring freedom from oppression.

- He will transform you into a giver.

- He will give you the desire and ability to meet and minister to people's needs.

- He will allow you to see yourself as you really are.

- God will give you spiritual insight and influence. No matter how dark and dismal the situation, your light will break forth like the dawn. You will help dispel the darkness and its power.

- Recovery and healing of various kinds may occur.

- Righteousness will precede you.

- The glory of God will be your protection and rear guard.

- God will answer your prayers. You will call and He will answer.

- God will manifest His presence with you. You will cry out and He will reply, "Here I am."

- He will adjust your attitude. Your gloom will become like midday.

- He will continually guide you.

- He will fulfill your desires in the midst of harsh and adverse circumstances.

- He will give you strength and energy.

- He will make you fruitful like a watered garden.

- He will make you like living water that never runs dry.

- You will become a rebuilder of right traditions and a godly heritage.

- You will become a restorer.

- You will become a repairer of breaches and gaps.

- God will lift you up and exalt you.

- He will give you more faith.

CORPORATE FASTING

Even as I have written about the biblical mandate of personal fasting, there's one other important issue that must be addressed—corporate fasting (the fasting and praying of an entire church or congregation). In the days ahead, I will be writing more about this additional opportunity in our churches. In the meantime, I pray that pastors and church leaders will come to recognize what "Forty Days of Spiritual Power" can do for the people of God as a whole. This program could be based on every member of the congregation fasting just one day a month, which would mean scores or even hundreds of Christians would be fasting every day for a full forty days.

The purpose of these forty days would be to involve individual Christians in fasting and prayer for the purpose of fulfilling the spiritual goals that churches believe God wants them to achieve. I'm confident that this all-church program could take any congregation to a higher level with God. Why is this program needed? Because individual Christians will seldom go any further than they are led to go in their walk with Christ.

It's my prayer that pastors and church leaders will be persuaded to consider such a program seriously in the days ahead.

SOME CONCLUDING REMARKS

I challenge you boldly and confidently to enter into the fullness of God's will and purpose for your life. True spiritual champions know that when Jesus Christ is not preeminent in their lives they will be open to failure and defeat. True spiritual champions give total allegiance to their Lord. Spiritual champions demonstrate absolute dependence on their Savior and a reckless abandonment to the authority and leadership of their Sovereign. Spiritual champions understand the privilege and responsibility of being children of the King. Human efforts will fail. Natural attempts will not satisfy. Ordinary tactics are finally reduced to mediocrity. There is no lasting contentment apart from God's will and His purpose for our lives. Unless we surrender completely to God's plan, we are destined to drift in a sea of disappointment, disillusionment, and depression. We are in constant need of supernatural power. Our only hope is in the life and love of our wonderful Lord, Jesus Christ.

Revival *will* come. Christians *will* be awakened. The world *will* be shaken from its catatonic complacency. You can take part and make a difference. "The difference you make *with* your life is contingent on the difference God makes *in* you. The difference you make in others will never be any greater than the difference which has been made in you by Jesus Christ. The dent we can make in our world will be insignificant without the power of Jesus Christ flowing through our lives."[1]

I encourage you to join with me and many others as we pray and fast for revival and renewal in our own lives, in our families, in our churches, and in our nation.

*"When you fast, put oil on your head and wash your face,
so that it will not be obvious to man that you are fasting,
but only to Your Father, who is unseen; and Your Father,
who sees what is done in secret, will reward you."*

MATTHEW 6:16–18

My Prayer and Fasting Journal

※

_____
_____
_____
_____
_____
_____
_____
_____
_____
_____
_____
_____
_____
_____
_____
_____
_____
_____
_____
_____
_____
_____
_____
_____

ENDNOTES

The Power of Prayer and Fasting

Chapter One

1. Boris Pasternak, *Doctor Zhivago* (New York: Pantheon Books Inc., 1958), 43.

Chapter Two

1. A. W. Tozer, "Entering the Holy of Holies": *Pulpit Helps*, July, 1996, p. 1.

2. *Revival Report*, February, 1994, 3.

Chapter Four

1. Max Lucado, *A Gentle Thunder* (Dallas: Word Publishing, 1995), 3–4.

Chapter Seven

1. Andrew Murray, *Great Evangelical Teaching: Absolute Surrender* (Nashville, Tenn.: Thomas Nelson, 1988), 718.

2. Bill Hybels, "Five Dangerous Prayers and Why You Should Pray Them": *Today's Christian Woman*, July/Aug., 1992, 41–43. Used by permission.

3. Oswald Chambers, *My Utmost for His Highest*, (New York: Dodd, Mead, and Co., 1935), 78.

Chapter Eight
1. Words: Latin, 6th century; translated M.F. Bell (1862–1947) Music: Erhaltus, Herr, melody from Geistliche Lieder, [543 #143: *The Hymnal 1982*; (Church Hymnal Corporation)]

2. Charles Swindoll, *Eternal Security: The Assurance of Our Salvation* (Grand Rapids, Mich.: Zondervan, 1995). Used by permission.

3. R.C. Sproul, *Before the Face of God, Book Two* (Grand Rapids, Mich.: Baker Book House, 1993), 116–17.

4. (Quoted in Seven Promises of a Promise Keeper, "A Man and His Family," James Dobson, 1994), 124.

Chapter Nine
1. James Dobson, *Hide or Seek* (Old Tappan, NJ: Fleming H. Revell, a division of Baker Book House, 1974, 1979), 13–14. Used by permission.

Chapter Ten
1. David B. Barrett analyzes "Mission Contact." *Decision*, May 1991, 21.

A Practical Guide
1. Ronnie W. Floyd, *The Meaning of a Man* (Nashville, Tenn.: Broadman and Holman Publishers, 1996), 11. Used by permission.